T0205416

Smart Innovation, Systems and Technologies

Volume 93

Series editors

Robert James Howlett, Bournemouth University and KES International,
Shoreham-by-sea, UK
e-mail: rjhowlett@kesinternational.org

Lakhmi C. Jain, University of Canberra, Canberra, Australia;
Bournemouth University, UK;
KES International, UK
e-mails: jainlc2002@yahoo.co.uk; Lakhmi.Jain@canberra.edu.au

The Smart Innovation, Systems and Technologies book series encompasses the topics of knowledge, intelligence, innovation and sustainability. The aim of the series is to make available a platform for the publication of books on all aspects of single and multi-disciplinary research on these themes in order to make the latest results available in a readily-accessible form. Volumes on interdisciplinary research combining two or more of these areas is particularly sought.

The series covers systems and paradigms that employ knowledge and intelligence in a broad sense. Its scope is systems having embedded knowledge and intelligence, which may be applied to the solution of world problems in industry, the environment and the community. It also focusses on the knowledge-transfer methodologies and innovation strategies employed to make this happen effectively. The combination of intelligent systems tools and a broad range of applications introduces a need for a synergy of disciplines from science, technology, business and the humanities. The series will include conference proceedings, edited collections, monographs, handbooks, reference books, and other relevant types of book in areas of science and technology where smart systems and technologies can offer innovative solutions.

High quality content is an essential feature for all book proposals accepted for the series. It is expected that editors of all accepted volumes will ensure that contributions are subjected to an appropriate level of reviewing process and adhere to KES quality principles.

More information about this series at http://www.springer.com/series/8767

Philippe J. Giabbanelli · Vijay K. Mago
Elpiniki I. Papageorgiou

Editors

Advanced Data Analytics in Health

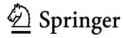 Springer

Editors
Philippe J. Giabbanelli
Computer Science Department
Furman University
Greenville, SC
USA

Elpiniki I. Papageorgiou
Department of Computer Engineering
Technological Educational Institute
Lamia
Greece

Vijay K. Mago
Department of Computer Science
Lakehead University
Thunder Bay, ON
Canada

ISSN 2190-3018   ISSN 2190-3026 (electronic)
Smart Innovation, Systems and Technologies
ISBN 978-3-030-08571-1   ISBN 978-3-319-77911-9 (eBook)
https://doi.org/10.1007/978-3-319-77911-9

Printed on acid-free paper

This Springer imprint is published by the registered company Springer International Publishing AG
part of Springer Nature
The registered company address is: Gewerbestrasse 11, 6330 Cham, Switzerland

Foreword

It is a curious feature of healthcare research and practice that solving each problem introduces new, more complex problems. In a century, we have extended human life by decades, overcoming the most devastating single-cause contributors to mortality through innovations such as antibiotics and vaccination. Yet, every solution, by extending human life, brings forward new maladies, often more complex in their nature. Progress in health care and various technological amenities now allow us to live shielded from the caprice of nature, surviving to old ages in which chronic and complex conditions from obesity and diabetes to cancer and depression are the major contributors to morbidity and mortality. This trend not only has increased the share of health research, innovation, and practice in the activities of our human societies but also has led to more complex problems dominating the landscape. The low-hanging fruits have largely been picked, and the emerging challenges are often complex conditions determined by a multitude of interacting causal factors spanning genes, cells, social norms, communities, and food supply chains, to name a few.

Fortunately, the rise in the complexity of health problems is matched by technological advances that have transformed the data and analysis landscape for researchers. Enhanced measurements tools, digital communication, and norms of openness in scientific community have been accelerating the availability of quantitative data informing health problems. In parallel, computational platforms and algorithms for making sense of these large datasets have been growing exponentially. These advances are promising for the ability of health research community to tackle the increasingly complex problems we face.

However, realizing this promise faces a bottleneck in our ability to stay abreast the relevant developments. Twenty years ago, a couple of graduate courses in (bio) statistics would have delivered an aspiring researcher to the forefront of analytical methods needed for most health research; today, it is challenging to even enumerate all the potentially relevant methods. Various promising tools are developed on a weekly basis, in fields as different as statistics, computer science, econometrics, and operations research, to name a few. Tracking relevant developments often requires identifying and reading single articles in disparate journals and using different terminologies, a challenging requirement for busy researchers often housed in disciplinary silos.

The current volume, edited by three talented researchers with complementary disciplinary expertise, provides a valuable resource to those of us interested to stay informed about the methodological advances in tackling complex health problems. The volume does an excellent job in identifying some of the more promising avenues for integrating advanced analytics into health research and offering informative introductions and examples. The four domains of data exploration, modeling and simulation, machine learning, and statistical analysis of case data offer a useful categorization of broad methodological domains that one may draw from. Within each domain two to three chapters introduce concrete methods and examples. The methods discussed are diverse, promising, and (previously) hard to learn in a single resource, a shortcoming that the current volume rectifies.

In reviewing the chapters, I was drawn to the clear exposition, the opportunity to learn more about various methods I had limited familiarity with, and the substantive insights on multiple fronts. For example, the chapter on dimensionality reduction not only provides a quick introduction to the methods for dimensionality reduction but also presents a software platform for data exploration using this method. Chapters "Navigating Complex Systems for Policymaking Using Simple Software Tools" and "Analyzing the Complexity of Behavioural Factors Influencing Weight in Adults" offer tools for analyzing, and examples of using, causal maps in understanding complex health topics such as obesity. The basic ideas in these chapters may not require much background, but the resulting tools can enhance the often unstructured way through which data from various stakeholders is integrated into an expert understanding of complex problems. The chapter on using agent-based models is noteworthy for rigorous use of empirical data along with a complex dynamic model, setting a laudable example for other dynamic modelers. Fuzzy cognitive maps (Chapters "Soft Data Analytics with Fuzzy Cognitive Maps: Modeling Health Technology Adoption by Elderly Women" and "Classifying Mammography Images by Using Fuzzy Cognitive Maps and a New Segmentation Algorithm") offer a flexible method for bringing qualitative data from stakeholder engagement and quantitative data together in a rigorous fashion; examples in technology adoption and image recognition provide testaments to the versatility of the method. Two other Chapters ("Machine Learning for the Classification of Obesity from Dietary and Physical Activity Patterns" and "Text-Based Analytics for Biosurveillance") introduce various machine learning methods including support vector machines, neural nets, discriminant analysis, and various steps and methods for text-based analytics. Each of these methods includes a large and growing literature, and the introductory chapters here can help researchers appreciate the basic ideas and promise of tools, and decide whether and how to learn more. The use of more standard statistical methods, such as difference-in-difference approach, combined with case studies in insurance expansion and integrated care exemplify the rigor needed for identifying causal impacts of interventions at community and organization levels. Finally, the book ends with an exploration of more novel topics such as smart home designs for elderly care and the architecture for working across different steps of genomic data acquisition and analysis. Beyond introducing specific methods, these chapters offer a great overview of related literature and methods, so that the reader can appreciate the landscape of analytical tools at one's disposal. Each chapter also includes a substantive contribution, spanning different domains, from obesity and hypertension to mammography and biosurveillance.

With its breadth and complementary contributions, this volume can be used in multiple ways. One can envision several chapters assigned as readings for graduate seminars introducing analytical tools for health research, or the book as a self-study resource for those interested to grasp an overview of the methodological landscape and get deeper in a few related tools. It can also act as a reference for occasional retrieval of material related to specific analytical methods. I hope that many readers will find this wealth of information as exciting as I have, and utilize this volume as they contribute to a better understanding and improvement of our health systems.

Cambridge, MA, USA   Hazhir Rahmandad
Albert and Jeanne Clear Career Development Professor
Associate Professor of System Dynamics
MIT

Preface

Data-driven decision-making is a long-established practice in the field of health, where the notion of "evidence base" is essential to identify, and subsequently argue for, specific interventions. As we now embrace the age of data science, the attention of both researchers and practitioners is shifting from traditional statistical methods for structured numerical datasets (e.g., spreadsheets) to new methods, types of data, and scale of analysis. In this edited volume, we cover all three aspects through the work of almost 50 scholars working at the intersection of computer science, engineering, public health, and biology.

Methods in data analytics are classified into three broad types. The first part of this volume is devoted to data *visualization* and exploratory methods, which can contribute to addressing common shortcomings across studies. For instance, a study may engage stakeholders (e.g., decision-makers and the broader community) only at the very beginning and at the very end of a project, which may be insufficient to capture the complexity of a context and identify acceptable solutions. In contrast, visualizations can provide an intuitive interface to engage stakeholders throughout a project, without requiring computational or statistical expertise. Visualizations are not limited to telling the story of a project and gathering feedback: They can also directly support scholars in interactively exploring the characteristics of their datasets. Chapters "Dimensionality Reduction for Exploratory Data Analysis in Daily Medical Research" and "Navigating Complex Systems for Policymaking Using Simple Software Tools" introduce and demonstrate key methods and software to explore medical and public health datasets. The second part focuses on Modeling and *Simulation*, and specifically predictive models in health. Such computational models are grounded in data analytics, as they make extensive use of data both for calibration and validation purposes. While they can serve many goals (e.g., identifying gaps in the data or illuminating key dynamics), Chapters "An Agent-Based Model of Healthy Eating with Applications to Hypertension" and "Soft Data Analytics with Fuzzy Cognitive Maps: Modeling Health Technology Adoption by Elderly Women" emphasize "what if" questions. What if we were to promote healthy eating: would it lower hypertension? What if we were to create new devices for health: would they be adopted by individuals? Models help us to project and evaluate the consequences of these actions. The third part concentrates on *Machine Learning*, which can be used on a variety of tasks including association rule learning (what relations exist between variables?) or clustering (what groups exist in the data based on measures of similarity?). Chapter "Machine Learning for the Classification of Obesity from Dietary and Physical Activity Patterns" provides an introduction to the task of classification, which builds a model from the samples currently available, and uses it to identify outcomes of interest for newer samples. Classification is further discussed in the subsequent chapters, as Chapter "Classifying Mammography Images by Using Fuzzy Cognitive Maps and a New Segmentation Algorithm" showcases how to integrate it with predictive models, while Chapter "Text-Based Analytics for Biosurveillance" points to the numerous ways in which classification supports the process of biosurveillance.

The types of data available for analysis have been historically diverse: textual accounts of one's medical conditions or images documenting the evolution of a case have existed well before the twenty-first century. The main novelty is our ability to efficiently utilize such types of data, alongside the more classical structured numerical datasets. This edited volume showcases the diversity of datasets that are now utilized in health studies. Standard statistical methods such as difference-in-difference are presented through case studies in Chapters "Young Adults, Health Insurance Expansions and Hospital Services Utilization" and "The Impact of Patient Incentives on Comprehensive Diabetes Care Services and Medical Expenditures". Chapters "Navigating Complex Systems for Policymaking Using Simple Software Tools" and "Analyzing the Complexity of Behavioural Factors Influencing Weight in Adults" discuss the collection and analysis of networked data, in which different drivers of a condition are connected based on causal relationships. This type of data also underlies the study in Chapter "An Agent-Based Model of Healthy Eating with Applications to Hypertension" (where social ties contribute to shaping health behaviors) and Chapter "Soft Data Analytics with Fuzzy Cognitive Maps: Modeling Health Technology Adoption by Elderly Women" (where the structure of the model is a causal map). Chapter "Classifying Mammography Images by Using Fuzzy Cognitive Maps and a New Segmentation Algorithm" details the process of image processing. Text data is the focal point of Chapter "Text-Based Analytics for Biosurveillance", which introduces the key steps of Natural Language Processing applied to automatic monitoring (i.e., surveillance).

The notion of "big data" is increasingly evoked when discussing the scale of analysis. The characteristics of big data are commonly referred to as the four V's (volume, variety, velocity, and veracity), with additional characteristics being proposed over the years (e.g., variability and value). To illustrate one of the challenges of big data, consider the following: we might have been able to build a model by doing several passes over the data, so the time it takes grows faster than the size of the data. When the size of the dataset becomes large, the time necessary may simply be prohibitive. This forces us to think in new ways (e.g., simplifying models and/or distributing the required computations), and explore alternative architectures (e.g., cloud computing). While several of these aspects are addressed throughout this edited volume, Chapter "Challenges and Cases of Genomic Data

Integration Across Technologies and Biological Scales" specifically addresses the challenges and benefits of working with very large datasets for biological discoveries in fields such as cancer research.

While the three facets of data analytics in health (methods, data types, and scale) have been individually covered in different books and reviews, we are pleased to present a volume that brings them all under one umbrella. This allows to highlight the synergies between these methods. For instance, classification in Chapters "Machine Learning for the Classification of Obesity from Dietary and Physical Activity Patterns"–"Text-Based Analytics for Biosurveillance" divides the data into a "training set" and a "testing set", so that a model is not evaluated on the data points used to build it. This same idea underlies the notion of "calibration" and "validation" used in the simulation models of Chapters "An Agent-Based Model of Healthy Eating with Applications to Hypertension" and "Soft Data Analytics with Fuzzy Cognitive Maps: Modeling Health Technology Adoption by Elderly Women". Emphasizing similarities and differences between methods allows scholars to navigate more fluidly between tools based on the specific needs of a project, rather than having to re-frame a project to fit with a single tool.

This edited volume is intended to be accessible to scholars interested in the methodological aspects of data analytics in health. Each chapter thus includes a comprehensive introduction and background for its approach. However, an exposition to current methods would not suffice to fully support the needs of scholars going forward. Consequently, this volume aims to match strong methodological foundations with a detailed understanding of how methods will need to change given the challenges in health. This is a common thread through the volume, as several chapters provide innovative methodologies, such as Chapter "Classifying Mammography Images by Using Fuzzy Cognitive Maps and a New Segmentation Algorithm" where the classic steps of image processing are augmented with simulation models. The last part is specifically devoted to new challenges and emerging frontiers. Chapter "The Cornerstones of Smart Home Research for Healthcare" examines the computational aspects of smart homes, which will be needed to cope with the aging of the population. This chapter extends the discussion in Chapter "Soft Data Analytics with Fuzzy Cognitive Maps: Modeling Health Technology Adoption by Elderly Women", where authors examine whether elderly women would use technology once it is developed. Chapter "Challenges and Cases of Genomic Data Integration Across Technologies and Biological Scales" highlights the benefits and technical difficulties in integrating datasets. Such integration allows to more accurately characterize phenomena over different temporal, spatial, or biological scales. However, there is a paucity of methods to work across scales and types of data, which will prompt methodological developments going forward. There are also challenges in the nature of scholarly work itself, as databases flourish or even compete but may not be maintained or remain consistent with each other.

Addressing such challenges will allow to better understand the causes and solutions to the many complex problems in health presented in this volume, ranging from cancer and obesity to aging.

Greenville, USA

Thunder Bay, Canada

Lamia, Greece

Philippe J. Giabbanelli
Assistant Professor
Vijay K. Mago
Associate Professor
Elpiniki I. Papageorgiou
Associate Professor

Contents

Part I
Data Exploration and Visualization

Dimensionality Reduction
for Exploratory Data Analysis
in Daily Medical Research

Dominic Giradi and Andreas Holzinger

Abstract In contrast to traditional, industrial applications such as market basket analysis, the process of knowledge discovery in medical research is mostly performed by the medical domain experts themselves. This is mostly due to the high complexity of the research domain, which requires deep domain knowledge. At the same time, these domain experts face major obstacles in handling and analyzing their high-dimensional, heterogeneous, and complex research data. In this paper, we present a generic, ontology-centered data infrastructure for scientific research which actively supports the medical domain experts in data acquisition, processing and exploration. We focus on the system's capabilities to automatically perform dimensionality reduction algorithms on arbitrary high-dimensional data sets and allow the domain experts to visually explore their high-dimensional data of interest, without needing expert IT or specialized database knowledge.

Keywords Dimensionality reduction · Visual analytics · Knowledge discovery

1 Introduction

The classic process of knowledge discovery in data (KDD) is a well known and meanwhile widely accepted process in the field of computer science and very important to create the *context* for developing methods and tools needed to cope with the ever growing flood of data [1] and the complexity of data. Particularly in the medical area we face not only increased volume and a diversity of highly complex, multi-dimensional and often weakly-structured and noisy data, but the pressing need for integrative analysis and modeling of data [2–4].

D. Giradi
RISC Software GmbH, Research Unit Medical Informatics, Linz University, Linz, Austria
e-mail: dominic.girardi@risc.uni-linz.ac.at

A. Holzinger (✉)
Holzinger Group, HCI-KDD, Institute for Medical Informatics/Statistics, Medical University Graz, Graz, Austria
e-mail: andreas.holzinger@medunigraz.at

© Springer International Publishing AG, part of Springer Nature 2018   3
P. J. Giabbanelli et al. (eds.), *Advanced Data Analytics in Health*, Smart Innovation, Systems and Technologies 93, https://doi.org/10.1007/978-3-319-77911-9_1

Fayyad et al. [1] define the process of knowledge discovery '*as the nontrivial process of identifying valid, novel, potentially useful, and ultimately understandable patterns in data*'. This process, which usually contains steps such as understanding the problem and data, data preparation, and data mining, is mostly performed by so called data scientists [5]. In this view the (biomedical) domain expert is rather put into a supervising, consulting and customer only role. In the HCI-KDD approach [6] this is different, as the domain expert takes on an active role and the goal is to integrate the expert directly into the machinery loop [7]. There is a need for easy-to-use data exploration system, mainly driven by the fact, that the analysis is done by domain experts, and not computer scientist [8].

It is very important to note that there is a huge difference between work-flows in biomedical research and clinical research, hence the KDD process in daily clinical research differs significantly from standard research work-flows. The role of the domain expert turns from a passive external supervisor—or customer—to an active actor of the process, which is necessary due to the complexity of the research domain [9]. However, these domain experts are now confronted with large amounts of highly complex, high-dimensional, heterogeneous, semi-structured, weakly-structured research data [10] of often poor data quality. The handling and processing of this data is known to be a major technical obstacle for (bio-)medical research projects [11]. However, it is not only the data handling that contains major obstacles, also the application of advanced data analysis and visualization methods is often only understandable for data scientists or IT experts. A survey from 2012 among hospitals from Germany, Switzerland, South Africa, Lithuania, and Albania [12] showed that only 29% of the medical personnel of responders were familiar with a practical application of data mining. Although this survey might not be representative globally, it clearly shows the trend that medical research is still widely based on standard statistical methods. One reason for the rather low acceptance rate is the relatively high technical obstacle that needs to be taken in order to apply often complex algorithms combined with the limited knowledge about the algorithms themselves and their output. Especially in the field of exploratory data analysis deep domain knowledge of the human expert is a crucial success factor.

In order to overcome some of the mentioned obstacles and to help to contribute to a concerted effort in dealing with increasing volumes of data, we present a generic, ontology-based data infrastructure for scientific research that supports the research domain expert in the knowledge discovery process; beginning with the definition of the data model, data acquisition and integration and acquisition, to validation and exploration. The idea is to foster a paradigm shift that moves the domain expert from the edge of the process to the central actor. The system is based on a generic meta data-model and is able to store the actual domain ontology (formal description of the research domain data structures) as well as the corresponding structured research data. The whole infrastructure is implemented at a higher level of abstraction and derives its manifestation and behavior from the actual domain ontology at run-time. The elaborated structural meta-information is used to reach a sufficiently high degree of automation in data processing, particularly for exploratory data analysis. This allows the domain experts to visualize more easily their complex and high dimensional research data. In this paper we present two different ontology-guided visualization methods: a parallel coordinate visualization and non-linear mapping visualization.

2 Related Research

The idea of using meta models to automatically create parts (data access layer, user interfaces) of data intensive software systems is a widely established method in model-driven engineering (MDE) [13], which is a promising approach to address platform complexity [14]. However, the MDE approach in general or concrete realizations such as the meta model-based approach for automatic user interface generation by da Cruz et al. [15]—just to provide an example—are used by software engineers to create source code or source code skeletons at development time. Our system derives the structure of the user interface from the meta model at run-time. There is no source code generation. From this perspective our system is related to the Margitte system by Renggli et al. [16]. Whilst the Margitte system is a general purpose framework, based on a self-describing meta-model, our system is based upon a meta-entity-relationship model—stored in a relational database—and clearly focused and specialized on scientific data acquisition and data processing considering the medical researcher as both a main user and administrator. There is a close relation to ontology-based systems: Zavaliy and Nikolski [17] describe the use of an ontology for data acquisition, motivated by the demand of adaptive data structures. They used an OWL (Web Ontology Language) [18] ontology to model their domain, which consists of four concepts (*Person*, *Hospital*, *Diagnosis* and *Medication*). However, there is no information given on user interface generation. Aside from this work, it was very hard to find any related work on absolutely generic ontology-based data acquisition systems. In most publications ontologies are used for information extraction from text [19–21], or to enrich the existing data with structural and semantic information, or to build a cross-institutional knowledge base. In [22] the authors describe the usage of ontologies for inter-hospital data extraction to improve patient care and safety by analyzing hospital activities, procedures, and policies. Here, the ontology is strongly connected to the project. In [23] e.g. the authors describe an ontology based system for extracting research relevant data out of heterogeneous hospital information systems. Here again, the purpose is to find a superior common data model to compare data of different medical institutions. The most comparable work was published in 2014 by Lozano et al. [24], who also present an ontology-based system, called OWLing. Their intention is comparable to the above-mentioned, but their implementation is completely based upon the web ontology-language OWL. The work of [25] is also based on OWL and uses inference and reasoning to support medical staff in pre-operative risk assessment. They use the ontology as knowledge base for decision support. Although its structure is adaptable, the absolute genericity is no objective of this project. Generally speaking, many of these projects use ontologies to store explicit domain knowledge and use this knowledge for inference, reasoning, and decision support—which is the fundamental idea behind ontologies: to make knowledge of the domain expert accessible to computer algorithms. Our approach aims in the opposite direction: we use ontologies to enable the domain expert to explore their complex, high-dimensional and voluminous research data on their own. The domain-ontology—holding structural and semantic information about the research data—allows the software to automatize many data processing operations and to provide guidance and assistance to the researcher. In this way, the technical obstacles which a non-IT user is confronted with, when he is working with complex data structures are reduced. The ontology-based approach allows domain-specific guidance and assistance on the one hand, while it guarantees domain-independence on the other hand. For applying the system in a completely different research domain only the domain-ontology needs to be (re-)defined, without changes to the software itself.

In this paper we concentrate on a particularly important aspect: Scientists working with large volumes of high-dimensional data are immediately confronted with the problem of dimensionality reduction: finding meaningful low-dimensional structures hidden in their high-dimensional observations—to solve this hard problem is a primary task for data analysts and designers of machine learning algorithms and pattern recognition systems [26]. Actually, we are challenged by this problem in everyday perception: extracting meaningful, manageable features out of the high-dimensional visual sensory input data [27].

The general problem of dimensionality reduction can be described as follows: Given the p-dimensional random variable $x = (x_1, \ldots, x_p)^T$, the aim is to find a representation of lower dimensions, $s = (s_1, \ldots, s_k)^T$ with $k < p$, which (hopefully) preserves the "meaning" of the original data. However, meaning is an human construct, same as "interesting", and is influenced by tasks, personal preferences and past experiences and many other environmental factors [28]. This makes it essential to put the domain expert into the loop of the knowledge discovery process [6], and to be aware of the important aspect that *feature extraction and feature transformation* is key for understanding data. The major challenge in KDD applications is to extract a set of features, as small as possible, that accurately classifies the learning examples [29]. Assuming n data items, each represented by an p-dimensional random variable $x = (x_1, \ldots, x_p)^T$, there are two types of feature transformation techniques: linear and non-linear.

In linear techniques, each of the $k < p$ components of the new transformed variable is a linear combination of the original variables:

$$s_i = w_{i,1}x_1 + \ldots w_{i,p}x_p, \quad \text{for} \quad i = 1, \ldots, k, \quad \text{or}$$

$$s = \mathbf{W}x,$$

where $\mathbf{W}_{k \times p}$ is the linear transformation weight matrix.

Expressing the same relationship as

$$x = As,$$

with $A_{p \times k}$, we note that the new variables s are also called the hidden or the latent variables. In terms of an $n \times p$ feature-document matrix X, we have

$$S_{i,j} = w_{i,1}X_{1,j} + \dots w_{i,p}X_{p,j}, \quad \text{for} \quad i = 1, \dots, k \quad \text{and} \quad j = 1, \dots, n$$

where j indicates the jth realization, or, equivalently,

$$S_{k \times n} = W_{k \times p}X_{p \times n},$$

$$X_{p \times n} = A_{p \times k}S_{k \times n}.$$

There are various methods how to attack this general problem, the two most known include: principal component analysis (PCA) and multidimensional scaling (MDS). PCA is the oldest and most known technique [30], and can be used in various ways to analyze the structure of a data set and to represent the data in lower dimension; for a classic application example see [31], and for details refer to [32]:

Tenenbaum et al. describe an approach for solving dimensionality reduction problems, which uses easily measured local metric information to learn the underlying global geometry of the data set, which is very different from classical techniques such as PCA and MDS. Their approach is capable of discovering the nonlinear degrees of freedom that underlie complex natural observations. In contrast to previous algorithms for nonlinear dimensionality reduction, the approach by Tenenbaum et al. efficiently computes a globally optimal solution, and moreover, for an important class of data manifolds, is guaranteed to converge asymptotically to the true structure [33].

3 Theoretical Background

3.1 Exploratory Visual Analytics

In contrast to statistical approaches aimed at testing specific hypotheses, Exploratory Data Analysis (EDA) is a quantitative tradition that seeks to help researchers understand data when little or no statistical hypotheses exist [34]. Often the exploratory analysis is rather based on visualization of the data than on descriptive statistic and other data mining algorithms. This graphical approach is often referred to as visual analytics. A scientific panel of the National Visualization and Analytics Center (a section of the Department of Homeland Security) defined visual analytics as the science of analytical reasoning facilitated by interactive visual interfaces [35]. Behind this rather technical definition Thomas and Cook provide a very practical view on the usage of visual analytics: End-users can apply visual analytics techniques to gain insight into large and complex data sets to identify the expected and to discover the unexpected [35]. Holzinger et al. [36] state, that one of the main purposes of such approaches is to gain insight into the data and to create new hypotheses. The central aspect of visual analytics is the integration of the human domain expert into the data analytics process. This allows to take advantage of his/her flexibility, creativity, and background knowledge and combine these skills with the increasing storage capacities and computational power of today's computers [37].

3.2 Parallel Coordinates

Parallel Coordinates are well known method for loss-free dimensionality reduction. Instead of arranging the axis of a coordinate system orthogonally—which is limited to two respectively three axis (two dimensional computer displays in a three dimensional world)—they are arranged in a parallel way. A point in a two dimensional orthogonal coordinate system is represented by a line in a multi-dimensional parallel coordinate system. In the context of parallel coordinates, this is known as the point-line duality. Parallel coordinates as a mean of computer-based data visualization of higher dimensions were introduced by Alfred Inselberg [38] from the 1980s up to now. Although parallel coordinates are known for some decades they are yet barely used in biomedical research [39]. On the other hand, their is an increasing number of publications on this raising from 14 in 1991 to 543 in 2011 on Google scholar [40], indicating the rising interest and relevance of this method.

3.3 Non-linear Mapping

Non-linear mapping is an application of multidimensional scaling (MDS). Multidimensional scaling is a method that represents measurements of similarity (or dissimilarity) among pairs of objects as distances between points of low-dimensional space [41]. Non-linear mapping extracts these measurements of dissimilarity from a data set in a high dimensional input space and subsequently uses MDS to scale them to a low-dimensional (usually two-dimensional) output space. In this way the high-dimensional topology of the input space is projected to the low-dimensional output space. A well known algorithm in this field is the Sammon's mapping algorithm by [42]. Sammon's mapping tries to reduce the error between the distance matrix in the high dimensional input space and the distance matrix of the low-dimensional output space, whereas the error E is defined as:

$$E = \frac{1}{\sum\limits_{i<j}[d_{ij}^*]} \sum\limits_{i<j}^{N} \frac{[d_{ij}^* - d_{ij}]^2}{d_{ij}^*}$$

The term d_{ij}^* refers to the distance of two data points i and j in the high-dimensional input space and d_{ij} refers to the distance of i and j in the low-dimensional output space. The initial position of the data points in the output space, thus the initial values of d_{ij} are chosen randomly. It is now up to the implementation how to minimize the error value. Sammon used a deepest descend method in his paper, but there are also other ways, like the Kohonen heuristic [43, p. 35].

4 Method

4.1 An Ontology-Centered Infrastructure

The basic assumption behind the ontology-centered data infrastructure is the modified role of the domain expert in the knowledge discovery process. In common definitions this role is characterized as customer-like, consulting role [5], the main part of the process is performed by a so called data analyst. In every day medical research it is often the domain expert himself who takes the leading role in this process and is then confronted with technical barriers regarding handling, processing, and analyzing the complex research data [11]. This is known to be a major pitfall to (bio-)medical research projects [44].

Based on this assumption we developed a data infrastructure for scientific research that actively supports the domain expert in tasks that usually require IT knowledge or support, such as: structured data acquisition and integration, querying data sets of interest by non-trivial search conditions, data aggregation, feature generation for subsequent data analysis, data pre-processing, and the application of advanced data visualization methods. It is based upon a generic meta data-model and is able to store the current domain ontology (formal description of the actual research domain) as well as the corresponding research data. The whole infrastructure is implemented at a higher level of abstraction and derives its manifestation and behavior from the actual domain ontology at run-time. Just by modeling the domain ontology, the whole system, including electronic data interfaces, web portal, search forms, data tables, etc. is customized for the actual research project. The central domain ontology can be changed and adapted at any time, whereas the system prevents changes that would cause data loss or inconsistencies.

The infrastructure consists of three main modules:

1. Management Tool: The Management Tool is the main point of interaction for the research project leader. It allows the modeling and maintenance of the current domain ontology, as well as data processing, data validation, and exploratory data analysis.

2. Data Interface: The data interface is a plug-in to the well established open source ETL (Extraction-Transform-Load) suite Kettle, by Pentaho. Kettle allows the integration of numerous data sources and enables the user to graphically model his ETL process. For the final step, the data integration into our system and ontology-based data-sink interface was implemented.

3. Web Interface: The web interface is an automatically created web portal, which allows the users—depending on their permissions—to enter, view and edit existing data records. It is usually used to manually complement the electronically imported data with information that was not available electronically (e.g. handwritten care instructions, fever graphs, etc.) or in an un- or semi-structured way (e.g. doctors letters, image data, etc.).

An essential module of the Management Tool is an ontology-guided expression engine. It interweaves grammatical and structural meta information and allows the users to graphically model expression on their data that can be used for feature generation, the definition of complex search queries or data validity rules.

For further details on the ontology-guided expression engine the reader is kindly referred to [45], and for further information on the system itself to [46] and [47].

4.2   Ontology-Supported Data Exploration

It is the underlying paradigm of the whole infrastructure to move the researching domain expert in the central role of the knowledge discovery process. While the system supports the user in necessary tasks like data integration and processing, the real benefit of the paradigm shift occurs in the step of visual data exploration. Here the elaborate domain knowledge of the expert together with the general capability of the human mind to identify patterns in visualizations and the computational power of novel algorithms and systems can be combined, as [39] state. The aim is to support the expert end users in learning to interactively analyze information properties thus enabling them to visualize the relevant parts of their data [48].

In terms of the the presented system, the exploratory data analysis takes place in the management tool. Here the user can query the data sets of interest and move them to a special area of the system, called the Exploration perspective. In contrast to the Data perspective, the data can not be deleted or manipulated—it is safe. It only can be removed from the current set of interest. This set of interest contains the selected records and by default all attributes these records have. The user can now easily remove unneeded attributes and create new ones by using the system's expression engine. The expression engine allows the user to aggregate data from all over the domain ontology data structures with one data set of interest. For each data set a standard report including descriptive statistics parameters and interactive histogram display can be shown. In here, data cleaning can be performed. Once the data set is cleaned and checked by the system's data validity engine, a number of data visualizations can be created automatically, ranging from simple scatter plots or histograms to parallel coordinates and non-linear mapping.

Ontology-Guided Visual Clustering It is an often re-occurring requirement in medical research to find groups of similar elements, e.g. patients with similar symptoms or anamnesis. This process is often referred to as clustering or unsupervised learning. Cluster analysis is defined as the organization of a collection of patterns (usually represented as a vector of measurements, or a point in a multidimensional space) into clusters based on similarity [49].

Cluster algorithms try to find groups of similar records and group them into meaningful clusters. The cluster membership of each data record is usually marked with a cluster number or cluster label. Without any visual check the result of the clustering is very hard to interpret. It provides no information on the shape of each cluster and no information of the topology among the clusters. Although cluster analysis is an established state-of-the-art methods, its direct benefit for the domain expert is very limited.

The most significant difference between supervised and unsupervised learning is the absence of a target value. Supervised learning algorithms try to minimize the error between a target value and a calculated value. Since the error is known, results of supervised learning algorithms can be evaluated. So it is possible to determine which algorithm yielded the best model. For clustering algorithms there is no error, no difference between calculated and desired values. So it is not possible to determine which is the best clustering. Moreover the quality of the result also depends on the user of the clustering, even if this understanding of quality stands in a contradiction to a calculated quality value [50].

While there is no gold standard to compare to, there a number of quality criteria for unsupervised learning algorithms. The sum-of-squared-errors criteria [51] is one of them, which is minimized by some clustering algorithms (e.g. the k-means algorithm). However, Fig. 1 shows up the limitations of those criteria. The data set itself doesn't show any obvious clustering. Three different cluster criteria were optimized for $c = 2$ (the number of clusters) and $c = 3$. All of these clusterings seem reasonable, there is no strong argument to favor one of them. While J_e (sum-of-squared-error criterion) tends to create two clusters of about equal size (for $c = 2$). J_d (determinant criterion [51] page 545) models two clusters of different sizes. Similar phenomena can be observed for $c = 3$ and the third criterion J_f (trace criterion [51] page 545). Although, there is no clustering with the data, the application of cluster algorithms would yield a number of clusters.

Furthermore, the result of some clustering algorithms may depend on a random initial state like k-means or the EM algorithm [52]. Some of the algorithms need the number of clusters as an input parameter. Although there are strategies to overcome these shortcomings, like the consensus clustering meta heuristic [53], the suitability for daily use of standard unsupervised learning algorithms is very limited.

In order to overcome these drawbacks of classical cluster algorithms the decision was made to follow the visual analytics paradigm also in the task of finding clusters. Therefore, the potentially high dimensional research data needs to be mapped

Fig. 1 One data set different criteria, different results [51]

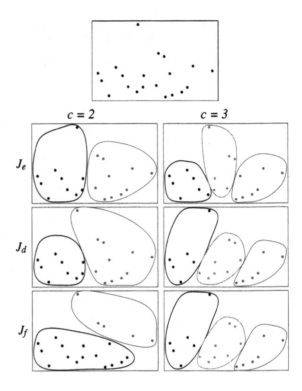

onto a two-dimensional display. Two well-known algorithms for this tasks are the Self-Organizing or Kohonen Map (SOM) [43] and the non-linear mapping algorithm Sammon's mapping [42]. Both algorithms try to minimize the error or mismatch between a topology in the n-dimensional source-space and the (mostly) two-dimensional target space. While the Kohonen Map yields a graph whose topology corresponds with the original topology, Sammon's mapping yields a cloud of dots, whereas each dot represents an input data record. In a theoretical evaluation [54] both algorithms were evaluated. Although the result of this evaluation preferred the SOM, practical tests with domain experts showed that the dot cloud was way easier to interpret than the network yielded by the SOM.

For the user, the non-linear mapping algorithm is hidden behind the notion 'Visual Clustering'. The only configuration, which is required by the user, is to select which attributes should be taken into account for the calculation of the distance or dissimilarity of two records. Then, the algorithm normalizes the data. Subsequently, a distance matrix is calculated, whereas for numerical variables an Euclidean distance is used and the Jaccard Metric [55] for categorical variables. Finally, the result is presented in a scatter plot. Via mouse wheel the user is able to change the variable that is used to color the dots. In this way, not only patterns in the topology of the data can be identified but also the correlation to other attributes according to the coloring.

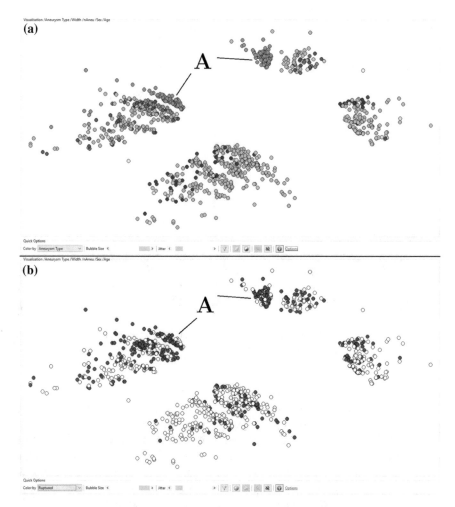

Fig. 2 An ontology-guided non-linear mapping of 1032 cerebral aneurysms with a distance calculation based on the following features: Aneurysm.Width, Aneurysm.Location, Patient.Number of Aneurysms, Patient.Age. **a** The aneurysms are colored according to their location. **b** The aneurysms are colored according to their rupture state: red are ruptured, white are none-ruptured [56]

Within the plot, the user is able to select data sets of interest and directly access and process the underlying data records.

Figure 2 shows the visualization of a real-world medical data set of 1032 cerebral aneurysms. A cerebral aneurysm is the dilation, ballooning-out, or bulging of part of the wall of an artery in the brain [57]. The data was collected using the previously described ontology-centered infrastructure, at the Institute for Radiology at the Campus Neuromed of the Medical University Linz. The parameters for the visual clustering were chosen by the medical experts. A more detailed description of the

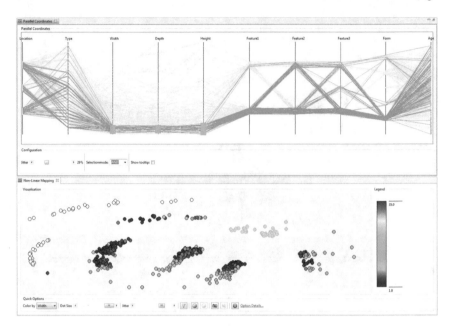

Fig. 3 A simultaneous display of a parallel coordinate system with a scatter plot showing the result of a non-linear mapping. The selection in the parallel coordinate system is highlighted (in green) in the scatter plot. Both visualization show the same data set as seen in Fig. 2

data set and the experiments can be found in [56]. The visualization revealed the high dimensional structure of the data set showing clusters of ruptured aneurysms (colored in red in Fig. 2—section *b*). When coloring parameter was switched to the location of the aneurysm (section *a* in Fig. 2), it was clearly visible that two of the previously seen clusters of ruptured aneurysms share the same location, which lead to the research-hypothesis that aneurysm in this location might be more prone to rupture. A hypothesis which turned out to be evident in medical literature [58]. Aside this confirmation and reproduction of already existing knowledge, the visualization yielded further interesting patterns which resulted in research hypotheses that are currently addressed by the medical researchers.

Plots showing the same set of interest are linked with each other in a way that the selection on one plot is automatically highlighted on all other plots as well. Figure 3 shows two linked displays of a parallel coordinate system and a visual clustering. The selection in the parallel coordinate system is highlighted in the scatter plot of the clustering.

Ontology-Guided Parallel Coordinate View Comparable to the visual clustering, the user is able to visualize any data set of interest in form of a parallel coordinate system. For this visualization no further configuration is required. The system automatically normalizes numerical attributes and maps categorical attribute to numeric ranges. By hovering the mouse over the axes the current numeric or the underlying categorical value are shown as a tool tip. Categorical and Boolean values can cause horizontal lines to overlap, which leads to the effect that the user is not able to distinguish whether there is only one record with a certain configuration or many. Therefore, a jitter slider was integrated into the visualization that adds a random off-set to values of Boolean and categorical attributes and let the corresponding lines drift apart. So it is perceptible if there are overlapping values. The selection within the parallel coordinate view is propagated throughout the system and highlighted in all other visualizations showing the same data set (see Fig. 3). Furthermore, selected records can be opened and edited, which allows the quick changing from data exploration to data revision or editing.

5 Conclusion

In this paper we presented an ontology-based research infrastructure, grounded in the central paradigm to put the researching domain expert in a central position of the knowledge discovery process. After supporting the researcher in data integration and handling, we now address the field of data exploration. Here, we chose a primarily visual approach using two completely different means of dimensionality reduction: parallel coordinates on the one hand, and non-linear mapping on the other. Both are well-known means of visualization in the field of computer science. However, our experiences showed that they are practically not used for medical research. Consequently, to lower the technical barrier to use this type of visualization algorithms, we use the structural meta-information of the central ontology, to reduce the configuration and pre-processing requirements to a minimum. The main advantages of our approach can be summarized by:

- Domain Independence: The presented software is completely domain independent and can be adapted to any research domain by modeling the central domain ontology. The whole system adapts to this ontology at run-time.
- Assistance to Domain Experts: The structural and semantic information from the domain ontology is used to actively support the domain expert—who is usually no IT-expert—in technically challenging tasks such as data integration, data processing and data analytics.
- Fully Integrated Visual Analytics: The described data visualization algorithms are seamlessly integrated into the system and can be applied to any given data set of interest. The necessary data pre-processing and the launching of the algorithms is automatized based upon the structural information from the domain ontology. All visualization allow the interaction and a direct drill-down to the underlying data.

Practical experiences within the clinical context demonstrated that medical researchers are surprised at a first glance that the visual clustering often yields properly separable clusters. They were not aware of the existence of subgroups in their patient collective and the question of correlation with the clusters to other attributes immediately arose, a question that could often be answered just by coloring the dots in the cloud, according to the desired attribute. Generally, the dot cloud, yielded by the visual clustering, proved to be interpretable without further explanation. According to our experiences, the parallel coordinate visualization often confuses end users the first time they are confronted with it. As soon as the first selection across the axis is performed and subsequently moved along the axis, the fundamental principle of the visualization get clear and invites researchers to quickly check their hypothesis by setting and moving selection markers along the axis.

There are also risks and limitations in visual analytics generally and of course in our approach specifically. Similarly to any data-based method the quality of the visualization strongly depends on the quality of the underlying data. Nevertheless, we recommend to have the first look on the original raw data, because there might be something "interesting" in it. Noisy or messy data yields meaningless or—even more dangerous—misleading visualizations and might lead to the danger of modelling artifacts [59]. To address this problem, the ontology based infrastructure supports a wide range of data quality and plausibility checks to increase data quality. Secondly, it is important for the users to understand that a visualization yields insights and hypotheses and not facts. Regarding the example which is shown in Fig. 2, it is very important to understand that the clearly visible connection between the ruptured aneurysm and their location is just a hypothesis. There is no prove for a (statistically significant) correlation or even a causality. Both need to be examined using statistics and further medical research.

6   Future Research

There are a number of further research activities planned along the presented infrastructure. At first, we will support the visual approach by a machine learning module. Comparable to the consensus clustering algorithm [53], where clustering algorithms in different settings are executed and their result is consolidated, a supervised learning meta-algorithm will be developed. The base hypothesis behind this idea is the following: when different supervised learning algorithms in multiple configurations are able to predict a certain target value, by using the selected features, there is most probably a (non-linear) correlation between the features and the target values. If all or most algorithms fail, then we have to assume, that there is no correlation—at least within the given data set. Here again, the main objective is to enable the researching domain expert to use advanced machine learning algorithms, hence to combine the computational and algorithmic power of the computer with the intelligence and experience of the domain expert.

Clustering algorithms are based on distance or dissimilarity measures. Currently, for categorical attributes the Jaccard metric is used. Although it is able to cope with multi-selectable categorical attributes, it does not take into account a possible similarity of the category enumeration values. Given two patients with each two diagnoses: Patient 1 suffers from a flu and has a broken shinbone, while patient 2 has a broken fibular and a pneumonia. A distance measure that ignores the similarity of flu and pneumonia, and broken shinbone and broken fibular returns a big dissimilarity between patient 1 and 2. With the knowledge that a flu and a pneumonia are very similar diseases and a broken shinbone is almost the same as a broken fibular, the two patients would be considered very similar. It is now subject to our current research to integrate this knowledge into the distance measures for clustering following the ideas of [60–62].

Currently, our system is designed to work with structured data. Unstructured data (e.g. free-text diagnoses, hand written care instructions, image data, etc.) can only be integrated into the system manually, using the automatically created web interface. For a more computer supported integration of electronically stored non-standardized (in medical jargon called: free text), an expansion and research in the field of information extraction is planned.

The system in its current state is suitable for storing highly structured data. It supports arbitrary complex and deep data structures. However, due to performance reason the number of attributes of each data class is limited. There is no fixed limit, however, keeping in mind performance and usability, it does not make sense to create more than 20 or 30 attribute to a class. This is an issue, when very high dimensional research data shall be integrated including genome expression data. Regarding the number of data sets the limiting factor is the performance of CPU respectively GPU of the user's machine. Especially the non-linear mapping has a very unfavorable runtime behavior. Experiments show acceptable performance up to several 10,000 of records with State-of-the-Art desktop PCs. Data sets with significantly higher number of data would require a preliminary sampling. For this kind of data special data storage and integration methods need to be found and future research will also focus on the integration of alternative visualization methods (e.g. [63, 64]), consequently our work provides several additional and alternative future research possibilities. A very important future issue is to foster transparency, i.e. to explain why a decision had been made [65].

References

1. Fayyad U, Piatetsky-shapiro G, Smyth P (1996) From data mining to knowledge discovery in databases. AI Magazine 17:37–54
2. Holzinger A, Dehmer M, Jurisica I (2014) Knowledge discovery and interactive data mining in bioinformatics—state-of-the-art, future challenges and research directions. BMC Bioinform 15:I1
3. Holzinger A (2017) Introduction to machine learning and knowledge extraction (make). Mach Learn Knowl Extr 1:1–20
4. Holzinger A, Malle B, Kieseberg P, Roth PM, Mller H, Reihs R, Zatloukal K (2017) Machine learning and knowledge extraction in digital pathology needs an integrative approach. In: Springer lecture notes in artificial intelligence volume LNAI 10344. Springer International, Cham, pp 13–50
5. Kurgan LA, Musilek P (2006) A survey of knowledge discovery and data mining process models. The Knowl Eng Rev 21:1–24

6. Holzinger A (2013) In: Human computer interaction and knowledge discovery (HCI-KDD): what is the benefit of bringing those two fields to work together? Springer, Berlin, Heidelberg, New York, pp 319–328
7. Holzinger A, Jurisica I (2014) Knowledge discovery and data mining in biomedical informatics: the future is in integrative. In: Interactive machine learning solutions. Springer, Berlin, Heidelberg, pp 1–18
8. Zudilova-Seinstra E, Adriaansen T (2007) Visualisation and interaction for scientific exploration and knowledge discovery. Knowl Inf Syst 13:115–117
9. Cios KJ, William Moore G (2002) Uniqueness of medical data mining. Artif Intell Med 26:1–24
10. Holzinger A, Stocker C, Dehmer M (2014) In: Big complex biomedical data: towards a taxonomy of data. Springer, Berlin, Heidelberg, pp 3–18
11. Anderson NR, Lee ES, Brockenbrough JS, Minie ME, Fuller S, Brinkley J, Tarczy-Hornoch P (2007) Issues in biomedical research data management and analysis: needs and barriers. J Am Med Inf Assoc 14:478–488
12. Niakšu O, Kurasova O (2012) Data mining applications in healthcare: research vs practice. Databases Inf Syst Balt DB&IS 2012:58
13. Frankel D (2003) Model driven architecture: applying MDA to enterprise computing. Wiley, New York
14. Schmidt DC (2006) Model-driven engineering. Computer 39:25–31
15. Cruz AMR, Faria JP (2010) A metamodel-based approach for automatic user interface generation. In: Petriu D, Rouquette N, Haugen A (eds) Model driven engineering languages and systems, vol 6394. Lecture notes in computer science. Springer, Berlin, Heidelberg, pp 256–270
16. Renggli L, Ducasse S, Kuhn A (2007) Magritte—a meta-driven approach to empower developers and end users. In: Engels G, Opdyke B, Schmidt D, Weil F (eds) Model driven engineering languages and systems, vol 4735. Lecture notes in computer science. Springer, Berlin, Heidelberg, pp 106–120
17. Zavaliy T, Nikolski I (2010) Ontology-based information system for collecting electronic medical records data. In: 2010 International conference on modern problems of radio engineering, telecommunications and computer science (TCSET), 125
18. McGuinness DL, van Harmelen F (2004) Owl web ontology language overview: W3c recommendation
19. Tran QD, Kameyama W (2007) A proposal of ontology-based health care information extraction system: Vnhies. In: 2007 IEEE international conference on research, innovation and vision for the future, 1–7
20. Holzinger A, Geierhofer R, Modritscher F, Tatzl R (2008) Semantic information in medical information systems: utilization of text mining techniques to analyze medical diagnoses. J Univers Comput Sci 14:3781–3795
21. Holzinger A, Schantl J, Schroettner M, Seifert C, Verspoor K (2014) Biomedical text mining: state-of-the-art, open problems and future challenges. In: Holzinger A, Jurisica I (eds) Interactive knowledge discovery and data mining in biomedical informatics, vol 8401. Lecture notes in computer science LNCS 8401. Springer, Berlin Heidelberg, pp 271–300
22. Kataria P, Juric R, Paurobally S, Madani K (2008) Implementation of ontology for intelligent hospital wards. In: Proceedings of the 41st annual Hawaii international conference on system sciences, 253
23. Kiong YC, Palaniappan S, Yahaya NA (2011) Health ontology system. In: 2011 7th international conference on information technology in Asia (CITA 11), 1–4
24. Lozano-Rubí R, Pastor X, Lozano E (2014) Owling clinical data repositories with the ontology web language. JMIR Med Inf 2:e14
25. Bouamrane MM, Rector A, Hurrell M (2011) Using owl ontologies for adaptive patient information modelling and preoperative clinical decision support. Knowl Inf Syst 29:405–418
26. Kaski S, Peltonen J (2011) Dimensionality reduction for data visualization (applications corner). IEEE Signal Process Mag 28:100–104

27. Holzinger A (2014) Trends in interactive knowledge discovery for personalized medicine: cognitive science meets machine learning. Intell Inf Bull 15:6–14
28. Beale R (2007) Supporting serendipity: using ambient intelligence to augment user exploration for data mining and web browsing. Int J Human-Comput Stud 65:421–433
29. Kalousis A, Prados J, Hilario M (2007) Stability of feature selection algorithms: a study on high-dimensional spaces. Knowl Inf Syst 12:95–116
30. Pearson K (1901) On lines and planes of closest fit to systems of points in space. Philos Mag 2:559–572
31. Hoover A, Jean-Baptiste G, Jiang X, Flynn PJ, Bunke H, Goldgof DB, Bowyer K, Eggert DW, Fitzgibbon A, Fisher RB (1996) An experimental comparison of range image segmentation algorithms. IEEE Trans Pattern Anal Mach Intell 18:673–689
32. Jackson JE (2005) A user's guide to principal components, vol 587. Wiley
33. Tenenbaum JB, de Silva V, Langford JC (2000) A global geometric framework for nonlinear dimensionality reduction. Science 290:2319–2323
34. Behrens JT, Yu CH (2003) In: Exploratory data analysis. Wiley
35. Thomas J, Cook K (2006) A visual analytics agenda. IEEE Comput Gr Appl 26:10–13
36. Holzinger A, Scherer R, Seeber M, Wagner J, Müller-Putz G (2012) Computational sensemaking on examples of knowledge discovery from neuroscience data: towards enhancing stroke rehabilitation. In: Information technology in bio-and medical informatics. Springer, 166–168
37. Keim DA, Mansmann F, Schneidewind J, Thomas J, Ziegler H (2008) Visual analytics: scope and challenges. Springer
38. Inselberg A (1985) The plane with parallel coordinates. The V Comput 1:69–91
39. Otasek D, Pastrello C, Holzinger A, Jurisica I (2014) Visual data mining: effective exploration of the biological universe. In: Interactive knowledge discovery and data mining in biomedical informatics. Springer 19–33
40. Heinrich J, Weiskopf D (2013) State of the art of parallel coordinates. STAR Proc Eurogr 2013:95–116
41. Borg I (1997) Modern multidimensional scaling: theory and applications. Springer, New York
42. Sammon JW (1969) A nonlinear mapping for data structure analysis. IEEE Trans Comput 18:401–409
43. Kohonen T (2001) Self-organizing maps, 3rd edn. Springer
44. Franklin JD, Guidry A, Brinkley JF (2011) A partnership approach for electronic data capture in small-scale clinical trials. J Biomed Inf 44(Supplement 1):S103–S108
45. Girardi D, Küng J, Giretzlehner M (2014) A meta-model guided expression engine. In: Intelligent information and database systems. Springer, 1–10
46. Girardi D, Arthofer K, Giretzlehner M (2012) An ontology-based data acquisition infrastructure. In: Proceedings of 4th international conference on knowledge engineering and ontology development, Barcelona, 155–160
47. Girardi D, Dirnberger J, Trenkler J (2013) A meta model-based web framework for domain independent data acquisition. In: The eighth international multi-conference on computing in the global information technology ICCGI 2013, 133–138
48. Holzinger A (2012) On knowledge discovery and interactive intelligent visualization of biomedical data-challenges in human-computer interaction & biomedical informatics. In: DATA
49. Jain AK, Murty MN, Flynn PJ (1999) Data clustering: a review. ACM Comput Surv 31:265–323
50. Elhawary M, Nguyen N, Smith C, Caruana R (2006) Meta clustering. Sixth IEEE Int Conf Data Min 1:107–118
51. Duda RO, Hart PE, Stork DG (2001) Pattern classification, 2nd edn. Wiley Interscience
52. Bradley PS, Fayyad UM (1998) Refining initial points for k-means clustering. In: Proceedings of the fifteenth international conference on machine learning, 91–99
53. Monti S, Tamayl P, Mesirov J, Golub T (2003) Consensus clustering: a resampling-based method for class discovery and visualization of gene expression microarray data. Mach Learn 52:91–118

54. Girardi D, Giretzlehner M, Küng J (2012) Using generic meta-data-models for clustering medical data. In: ITBAM, Vienna, 40–53
55. Boriah S, Chandola V, Kumar V (2008) Similarity measures for categorical data: a comparative evaluation. Red 30:3
56. Girardi D, Küng J, Kleiser R, Sonnberger M, Csillag D, Trenkler J, Holzinger A (2016) Interactive knowledge discovery with the doctor-in-the-loop: a practical example of cerebral aneurysms research. Brain Info 3:133–143
57. NIH: Cerebral aneurysm information page (2010)
58. Bijlenga P, Ebeling C, Jaegersberg M, Summers P, Rogers A, Waterworth A, Iavindrasana J, Macho J, Pereira VM, Bukovics P et al (2013) Risk of rupture of small anterior communicating artery aneurysms is similar to posterior circulation aneurysms. Stroke 44:3018–3026
59. Wartner S, Girardi D, Wiesinger-Widi M, Trenkler J, Kleiser R, Holzinger A (2016) Ontology-guided principal component analysis: reaching the limits of the doctor-in-the-loop. In Renda EM, Bursa M, Holzinger A, Khuri S (eds) Proceedings of 7th International conference on information technology in bio- and medical informatics, ITBAM 2016, Porto, Portugal, 5–8 Sept, 2016. Springer International Publishing, Cham, pp 22–33
60. Hsu CC (2006) Generalizing self-organizing map for categorical data. IEEE Trans Neural Netw 17:294–304
61. Boutsinas B, Papastergiou T (2008) On clustering tree structured data with categorical nature. Pattern Recognit 41:3613–3623
62. Gibert K, Valls A, Batet M (2014) Introducing semantic variables in mixed distance measures: impact on hierarchical clustering. Knowl Inf Syst 40:559–593
63. Lex A, Streit M, Kruijff E, Schmalstieg D (2010) Caleydo: design and evaluation of a visual analysis framework for gene expression data in its biological context. In: 2010 IEEE pacific visualization symposium (PacificVis), IEEE, pp 57–64
64. Mueller H, Reihs R, Zatloukal K, Holzinger A (2014) Analysis of biomedical data with multilevel glyphs. BMC Bioinf 15:S5
65. Holzinger A, Plass M, Holzinger K, Crisan GC, Pintea CM, Palade V (2017) A glass-box interactive machine learning approach for solving np-hard problems with the human-in-the-loop. arXiv:1708.01104

Navigating Complex Systems for Policymaking Using Simple Software Tools

Philippe J. Giabbanelli and Magda Baniukiewicz

Abstract Comprehensive maps of selected issues such as obesity have been developed to list the key factors and their interactions, thus defining a network where factors (e.g., weight bias, disordered eating) are represented as nodes while causal connections are captured as edges. While such maps contain a wealth of information, they can be seen as a maze which practitioners and policymakers struggle to explore. For instance, the Foresight Obesity Map has been depicted as an 'almost incomprehensible web of interconnectedness'. Rather than presenting maps as static images, we posit that their value can be unlocked through interactive visualizations. Specifically, we present five required functionalities for interactive visualizations, based on experimental studies and key concepts of systems thinking in public policy. These functionalities include shifting from simple 'policy inputs' to loops, capturing what unfolds between an intervention and its evaluation, and accounting for the rippling effects of interventions. We reviewed ten software that support different policy purposes (visualization, argumentation, or modeling) and found that none supports four or all five of the functionalities listed. We thus created a new open-source software, `ActionableSystems`. The chapter details its design principles and how it implements the five functionalities. The use of the software to address policy-relevant questions is briefly illustrated, taking obesity and public health nutrition as guiding example. We conclude with open questions for software development and public health informatics, emphasizing the need to design software that supports a more inclusive approach to policy-making and a more comprehensive exploration of complex systems.

P. J. Giabbanelli (✉)
Computer Science Department, Furman University, Greenville, SC 29613, USA
e-mail: giabbanelli@gmail.com

M. Baniukiewicz
Department of Computer Science, Northern Illinois University, DeKalb, IL 60115, USA
e-mail: z1791304@students.niu.edu

© Springer International Publishing AG, part of Springer Nature 2018   21
P. J. Giabbanelli et al. (eds.), *Advanced Data Analytics in Health*, Smart Innovation,
Systems and Technologies 93, https://doi.org/10.1007/978-3-319-77911-9_2

1 Introduction

> As we enter an era marked by more complex drivers of population health and by diseases with multifactorial roots [...], it will be more useful to have in our population health armamentarium the capacity to model the potential impacts of different manipulations of the multiple factors that produce health. (Galea et al. [1])

Studies at the intersection of systems science and population health have demonstrated the usefulness of computational models for conditions driven by multiple interacting factors. For example, agent-based models of obesity have allowed to reconcile peer influences on food and physical activity behaviors with environmental (e.g. built environment) and individual (e.g. stress and depression) factors [2–4]. Such models are particularly useful for policymaking, as they allow to evaluate the health impacts of complex interventions [5], or can answer 'what-if' (also called 'what happens if') scenarios [1] in which policymakers explore the consequence of several policy levers either independently or in a synergistic fashion. Given the support that computational models can offer, they have become an increasingly popular tool in public health. In the case of obesity, there were only a handful of models in the 2000s [6, 7] but the recent years have seen so many models that they were the subject of several dedicated reviews [8, 9].

The emphasis in a computational model has historically been to capture the salient characteristics of a phenomenon. For instance, our early model of obesity focused on environmental and peer influences on changes in body weight. It thus had to capture how peers and the environment come together in affecting one's physical and food behaviors, which in turn can affect one's weight depending on physiological factors (e.g. metabolic rate) [3]. Policy levers are limited to a subset of variables in the model: the gender or metabolism of individuals cannot be changed by policies, but social norms may be amenable to changes [10, 11]. Running 'what-if' scenarios then consists of assigning different values to these variables, either independently (which is common yet statistically inefficient) or using Design of Experiments techniques [12]. We recently discussed two issues with this approach to 'what-if' scenarios [13]. First, policy levers may not be independent. For example, a high density of restaurants might lead to increased market competition in part through larger portion sizes. A 'what-if' scenario may artificially set values for density of restaurants and portion size, without realizing that the value taken by one affects the other. Second, a policy is not merely an abstract concept: it eventually has to be implemented by coordinating across sectors or jurisdictional boundaries. This involves many stakeholders, which have to work at different time scales. Consequently, inputs to a model may not be directly set to a value but instead change gradually, at different speeds for different inputs. In sum, rather than freely manipulating a collection of disparate inputs, policy-relevant models should include the essential interactions between inputs. This can be achieved by adding another *layer* to models, which captures the interactions between inputs for policy purposes. Any 'what-if' scenario would be done in this layer, and then passed to the model [13]. Since interactions between pairs of

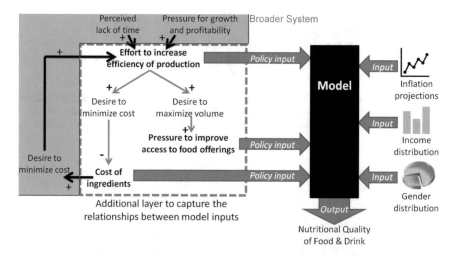

Fig. 1 A policy may be targeting three inputs of a model (efficiency of production, access to food offerings, cost of ingredients). Using the relevant part of the Foresight Obesity Map, we can include the relationships between these inputs in a layer separate from the model (dashed frame). Relevance is a matter of model boundaries, as the map offers a very broad perspective (light blue)

factors define a network, we use the term 'layer' to refer specifically to the network connecting the inputs of a policy-relevant simulation model.

There are four essential requirements in driving a policy-relevant model through a layer accounting for inter-dependencies between the model's inputs. First, we need to *develop the layer*, that is, the set of relationships between inputs along with relevant metadata (e.g., causal strength or time scales). This may be done from scratch. Alternatively, very large systems have already been *mapped*: for instance, in obesity research, the Foresight Obesity Map provides a comprehensive overview of relationships between factors related to weight or well-being. One may thus tease out the right part of such maps to construct the layer (Fig. 1), instead of starting from scratch. Despite the existence of many such maps, difficulties include (i) the lack of a comprehensive database or repository to find a map for a specific population health context, (ii) the wide range of quality or level of trust in existing maps, and (iii) the use of very different techniques to produce maps.[1]

Second, the development of the layer should *include relevant stakeholders* such as policymaker(s) or community member(s), whose views should shape which inputs are modified in 'what-if' scenarios and which outputs are monitored. Third, the layer needs to be *connected to the model*. This connection may not be trivial, as discussed elsewhere [20–22].

---

[1] Causal networks are formed of directed weighted relationships [14, 15], to which Fuzzy Cognitive Maps add an inference engine allowing to simulate the consequences of these relationships and thus test their validity [16, 17]. System Dynamics go even beyond, by including time effects and lags [18, 19].

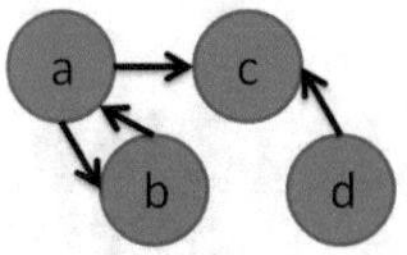

	a	b	c	d
a	0	1	1	0
b	1	0	0	0
c	0	0	0	0
d	0	0	1	0

Fig. 2 A *node-link* diagram (left) shows each factor as one node, and the connections between nodes as arrows. The shapes around the factors can omitted to only leave the factors' names. A different category of visualization for the same data is a *matrix* (right), which is not used here

During all these steps, the challenge is to *navigate the layer*. This challenge is the focus of the present chapter. Our usability study with policymakers in British Columbia (Canada) found that navigating even a medium-size policy layer (shown as node-link diagram in a typical network visualization; Fig. 2 can be a much more demanding task than handling seemingly disconnected inputs [23]. The Foresight Obesity Map exemplifies the difficulty of showing a system to stakeholders using a node-link diagram visualization. As pointed out in Hall et al. [24] (emphasis added), "the *complexity* of the obesity epidemic is graphically illustrated by the *web* of interacting variables". This is echoed by Siokou et al. [25]:

> With 100 or so causal factors, and 300 or more connections linking each cause to one or more of the others, the Foresight diagram is a complicated, almost incomprehensible web of interconnectedness that depicts the drivers of obesity prevalence and the ways in which they depend on each other. The diagram is brilliantly useful in demonstrating the complexity of factors driving the current obesity trend, but the scale and number of interactions in the diagram make it difficult to see how one might use it in any practical way to develop systemic approaches to obesity prevention.

Our aim is to support stakeholders in navigating complex maps, such that existing ones (e.g., Foresight Obesity Map) can be used as guidance tools for the design of policies rather than as symbols of complexity. Our main contributions in this chapter are as follows:

- Building off an existing map leads to higher cognitive complexity (more concepts and connections) but the upshot is a better informed, less ad-hoc policy layer. We identify the key functionalities that software need to improve the grounding of policy in scientific data, and we implement these functionalities as the new open-source `ActionableSystems` software.
- Being overwhelmed by complexity is a well-known problem encountered not only by participants but also by modelers. Our work on better navigating complex maps thus also helps modelers.

The next section presents five required functionalities, grounded in experimental studies and key concepts of systems thinking in public policy. Then, we contrast these functionalities with those supported in existing software for visualization, argumentation, or modeling. Having identified unique needs for a new software, we introduce our open-source solution `ActionableSystems` in Sect. 3. A brief demonstration is given in Sect. 4, with additional examples at https://youtu.be/OdKJW8tNDcM. Finally, we briefly discuss research directions in public health informatics, and we provide concluding remarks.

2 Functionalities to Navigate Maps with a Policy Focus

2.1 Knowledge Management

A wealth of information may be available about a given system. As pointed out by Dorner, this leads to an "informational overload" [26, p. 88]. In our previous study, we asked policymakers to provide their overall thoughts on a software supporting the use of maps for policymaking. Our thematic analysis revealed that participants did not see the role of software as limited to exploring or planning: they also thought about the potential to address the overload issue. They suggested that the software could serve as a tool for evidence synthesis: in the words of a participant, "if I could just go to one place, it would have all the information, that's sort of my dream" [23]. Organizing information serves multiple purposes. First, it can help to justify policies. Second, it provides a platform for knowledge integration and communication. Given the multi-sectoral nature of public policies, factors in a map may have different (or no) meanings for different stakeholders. This is exemplified by our map for obesity and well-being [15], which included physiological (e.g., adipocytes, inflammation), legal (e.g., restrictive covenants), and behavioral factors (e.g., disordered eating, eating disorder). A software can thus support the annotation of maps to clarify the meaning of each term, and possibly synthesize current knowledge about the term. Third, only having the name of a factor without contextualization can be problematic: "deconditionalizing abstractions are dangerous. The effectiveness of a measure almost always depends on the context within which the measure is pursued" [26, p. 95].

Functionality #1: Participants need to access and update the definitions and evidence supporting each factor.

In the same theme of facilitating data integration and communication, a new software should account for the existing workflow as participants should be able to make sense of existing data (from prior work) and integrate the software with tools commonly used in their area of expertise. In short, we need integration with existing tools. Research on Information and Communication Technology (ICT) to support policies has shown that many categories of tools exist, and within each, many tools are available [27]. The three categories with which the proposed software would directly integrate are visualization (which serve for information provision), argumentation (which support structured deliberation), and simulation tools (which address 'what-if' questions through computations). There are also different forms of integration. For example, scientific workflow systems can connect applications in pipelines where they automatically exchange information. The emphasis here is not on the automation but on supporting human decision-making processes, thus a new software should at least be able to take in data created via other tools.

Functionality #2: Participants need to manually exchange information between the new software and existing visualization, argumentation, and simulation tools.

2.2   Cognitive Limitations

The idea of an 'input' to a model is often rooted in a simple cause/effect reasoning: a change in one of the input factors triggers a changes in the model, which are reflected in a *different* set of factors labeled as outputs. As there is a "tendency to think in terms of isolated cause-effect relationships" (p. 34), this conceptualization of an input is commonly held [26]. In contrast, systems science and systems thinking emphasize the importance of loops:

> What really differentiates this kind of thinking from ordinary linear cause/effect reasoning is that none of these concepts can be regarded as more primary than the other. A change can be initiated everywhere in an event circle and after a certain time be read off as either cause or effect elsewhere in a system [28].

In this perspective, an 'input' is simply a part of the system selected for a policy intervention. A change in the input may trigger self-regulating mechanisms in the system, which eventually affect the input itself. Such mechanisms are well illustrated for complex conditions such as obesity (Fig. 3) through the Foresight Obesity Map, or the landmark *Thinking in Circles About Obesity* [29]. When considering whether a functionality is required, it should not only be an important feature, but one that participants need assistance with. The volume *Structure of Decision: the cognitive maps of political elites* examined how participants thought of systems, and whether they were aware of existing loops. Throughout the book, findings are consistent: participants did not show that they were thinking of loops when discussing complex systems. Ross saw it as peculiar that "those who set policy think only acyclically, especially since the cyclical nature of causal chains in the real world has been amply demonstrated" [30]. Examinations showed that the odd lack of loops or feedbacks in the maps was not due to lacking expertise, voluntarily simplifying the structure, of being focused on the near-term. Rather, the suggestion was to look for a cognitive explanation [31]: individuals unconsciously reduce complexity [32]. Therefore, loops have been shown to be crucial in understanding a complex system, and users need support to navigate them.

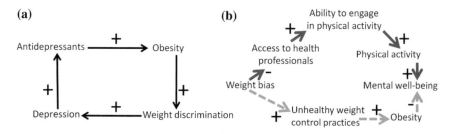

Fig. 3 Example of a loop in obesity (**a**), where some classes of antidepressants cause weight gain [3]. Example of disjoint paths from weight bias to mental well-being (**b**), going through physical activity (solid red arrows) or eating behavior (dashed blue arrows)

> Functionality #3: Participants need to easily find the loops such that they can think of policy 'inputs' within the context of a broader system.

Similarly to loops, other patterns in the map are relevant to policies and difficult to manage. A policy intervention may target some factor(s) and measure its impact on other(s). In between, there can be disjoint paths carrying the intervention (Fig. 3). For example, the intervention may fail significantly in one path and mask the relative success of another path. Understanding how the intervention permeates through the system is thus important for its evaluation. Disjoint paths face the same issue as loops: individuals reduce complexity and ignore multiple paths [32]. According to Dorner, omissions are one of the multiple reasons for failure in decision-making processes [26, p. 189]: it is essential to identify and analyze events developing within the system, and particularly the ones emerging as a side effect of our actions. Seeing all paths connecting two factors, rather than the one path which we may have monitored, may thus limit omissions.

> Functionality #4: Participants need to easily find disjoint paths, in order to monitor how interventions unfold between a starting point and the outcomes.

Finally, the design and evaluation of an intervention may have taken into account what gets directly affected by the policy, the outcomes, and everything in between (through disjoint paths). However, a long-established hallmark of systems thinking is to understand "the rippling effects created by choices" [33], even if the effects do not contribute to the outcome. For instance, the ecological model of health promotion posits that (emphasis added) [34]:

> individual, familial, communal, national, international, and global health is highly intertwined and interdependent. Negative perturbations in any of the functional units may have untold negative *rippling effects*

Note that the goal should not be to see *all* rippling effects. In some maps, an intervention may impact a massive number of factors, and it would be overwhelming rather than instructive to see them all. Rather, participants should be able to access a *filtered* set of rippling effects, depending on their needs. There are many possible needs: participants may want to ensure that a given set of factors are not affected by the policy (preserving a status-quo), sort the factors that are affected into categories (for cross-sectorial coordination), or perform an exploratory search with a limited depth (to see what would be affected through paths of up to x factors).

Selecting one variable as central is a common analytical approach. However, one should be cautious when anchoring a system around a given variable, as it may give a misleading feeling of control or prompt the analyst to take a reductionist approach [26, pp. 186–188]:

> If everything else depends on [the central variable] anyway, we dont have to worry about the status of other variables. We can also focus our planning on the one core variable. [...] If we develop a reductive hypothesis and see everything as dependent on a central variable, we not only make things easier, we also derive the reassuring feeling that we have things under control. [...] Forming simple hypothesis and limiting the search for information shorten the thought process and allows a feeling of competence.

Functionality #5: Participants need to find and filter the rippling effects of interventions.

2.3   Functionalities Supported by Existing Software

There exists plethora of software for visualization, argumentation, or modeling. As a comprehensive analysis of these software and their reviews would be the subject of a dedicated review, we instead focus on a subset of these software drawing from a recent comparative analysis [27]. In Table 1, we summarized whether these software support the five functionalities defined in the previous section.

Out of ten software, we found that loops were only supported by the software Vensim, and similarly only the software Gephi provided (limited) support to finding paths. In this case, it allowed to find the *shorter* paths, instead of *all* paths that lead to a selected outcome. The other functionalities were supported by more software. Rippling effects were supported in two software, with Vensim allowing to see rippling effects on all the system (i.e., without filtering) and Commetrix offering an advanced level of customization including the depth. Note that to qualify as rippling effects, we looked for a depth greater than 1: simply clicking on a node and see what it *directly* affects was not counted as supporting *rippling* effects.

Many software offered the possibility of storing definition and evidence, but varied tremendously in how convenient they make it for users to access or update the data. In Gephi and Visone, data about factors and their relationships is imported in the form of a spreadsheet, so users 'could' go through the internal data storage and manually create/edit columns for meta-data on definitions and supporting evidence. In Health Infoscape and MentalModeler, the access is much more immediate: clicking on a factor suffices to see the information as either a pop-up window (in `Health Infoscape`) or a side panel with notes (in `MentalModeler`). Finally, all software but two allowed to import and export files. However, the intention is not to merely to have a large collection of formats, but to promote interoperability between software such that practitioners can add capabilities to an existing workflow. Findings on formats are thus nuanced: three software operate with their own formats (`iThink`, `Vensim`, `MentalModeler`), two are meant for graphs yet they each use over ten different formats (`Gephi` and `Visone`), and even the same file CSV extension is used to store very different graph data (one list for `Gephi` but two lists in `Commetrix`, and a matrix in `Visone`). This paints some of the difficulties that practitioners have in navigating this software ecosystem, with its many formats, and even different meanings for what could appear to be the same format.

In summary, no software supports 4 or all 5 of the key functionalities for systems thinking in policymaking. Only `Commetrix` fully supports 3 functionalities, while `Vensim` and `Gephi` partially support 3. As the need for software supporting all functionalities is currently unmet, the next section details the design of our solution.

We note that the software surveyed here also have their own strengths, which are not necessarily captured by the five functionalities on which we focus. While a software may not easily connect to others through file input/output, some provide additional (often less intuitive) means to facilitate a workflow. `Visone` possesses a console to use the language R, which offers extended capabilities to connect with other software. `Gephi` is designed as an extensible software (i.e., uses a plug-in architecture), with over 21 plugins to import and export. A visualization software also tends to provide extensive support for different ways to render information. In the case of a map, the position of the map elements on the screen is determined by a *layout*, and software often support a variety of layouts (with over 15 layouts in `Gephi` and over 10 in `Visone`). Even though the modeling software studied here all deal with some extension of the concept of graphs, none supports layouts: the user is entirely responsible for deciding on the position of all elements. Their strength is instead to support practitioners in quantitatively evaluating what-if scenarios.

3 Proposed Software: `ActionableSystems`

3.1 Overview

The design of our proposed software took place over a three year period. Starting in 2015, our joint work with the Provincial Health Services Authority (PHSA) of British Columbia produced a very comprehensive policy map [15], which was difficult to analyze with existing software (Table 1). Through extensive discussions with members of the PHSA and other researchers, we developed a software tailored to the PHSA map. In 2016, we pilot-tested the software with several policymakers [23]. Our usability sessions resulted in over 30 recommendations on how

Table 1 Current ICT software and the five key functionalities

Software	Definitions and evidence	Formats	Loops	Paths	Rippling effects
Gephi	Embedded in the data (spreadsheet)	Imports: 11 formats including GraphML, Pajek, UCINET, and CSV (edge list or matrix). Exports: 6 formats including CSV and GraphML	No (attempted a plugin but does not work)	Yes, shortest paths only	No
Visone	Embedded in the data (spreadsheet)	Imports: GraphML, CSV/TXT (adjacency matrix), UCINET, Pajek, edge list, Siena. Exports: GraphML	No	No	No
Commetrix	Yes	Imports: Excel, XML, database (mySQL). Exports: CSV (node and link files)	No	No	Yes, with advanced filtering
Gapminder	No	No imports. No exports	No	No	No
Health Infoscape	Yes, available when clicking on a factor	Developed for one dataset only. No exports	No	No	No
Google Public Data Explorer	No	Imports: public data from Google or ones dataset. No exports	No	No	No
MentalModeler	Yes, as side notes	Imports: own format (MMP). Exports: MMP, CSV	No	No	No

(continued)

Table 1   (continued)

Software	Definitions and evidence	Formats	Loops	Paths	Rippling effects
iThink	The user can add a text area to the model	Imports: own formats (STMX, ITMX), system dynamics model (XMILE)	No	No	No
Vensim	No	Imports: own formats (MDL, VMF, VPM)	Yes	No	Yes, without filtering
CLASPs Policy Analysis Modeling Systems (PAMS)	Yes, in Excel cells	Designed for Excel workbooks	No	No	No

to improve the user experience. In addition, the analysis of semi-structured interviews revealed that policymakers saw more potential uses for the software than it was initially designed for. Based on these results, we clarified the key functionalities that policymakers need to navigate policy maps (Sect. 2), and we created the new ActionableSystems software focused on these functionalities. Our software is written in the Java programming language and is open-source. It is hosted on the third-party repository Open Science Framework at https://osf.io/7ztwu/, where programmers can re-purpose the code, while users can download and run the software.

3.2   Design Principles

Three principles underlie the design of ActionableSystems. First, the software should be *simple*. The expertise of our intended users resides in policymaking, or in specific domains impacted by a policy. We do not assume that users are experts with specific computer techniques, such as node-diagram visualization. Consequently, the software needs (i) to use a language that is free of technical jargon, (ii) contextualize what its functionalities mean in a policymaking context, and (iii) include training. Figure 4 illustrates these principles. The left panel uses simple terms (e.g., 'See' instead of 'Interactive Visualization') and operations emphasize what they are for rather than how they work (e.g., the button "Cant see well? Click here to reorganize!" would be labeled as applying a network layout in many software). Examples are provided in three forms: long walkthrough tutorials (accessed via the 'Tutorials' button), legends (Fig. 4, bottom left), and tool-tips (e.g., hovering over a policy domain provides examples of what it includes).

Our second principle is to emphasize *consistency*. This is a key principle in design, and it contributes to making a software intuitive to use. It requires that similar elements are seen the same way, and that similar controls function the same way. For example, simple elements such as buttons in the same category should have the same sizes and fonts: Fig. 4 shows visual consistency for the main buttons in the left panel, sub-categories in the top panel, and tool-specific buttons in the bottom panel. One added difficulty in maintaining visual consistency in our software is that the same data can be viewed in different ways, each emphasizing a different aspect: the policy map can be seen at a high level (Fig. 4), or through specific cycles and disjoint paths. All these views maintain visual consistency on some aspects (e.g., the thickness of a causal relationship shows its strength) but differ on others (e.g., relationships are arranged in a circle when showing a cycle). Consistency in control is relatively easier to maintain, as interactions within a same category such as 'See' all trigger the same effect (e.g., a double-click always packs or unpacks a policy domain into its individual factors).

Finally, our third principle is *relevance*. Our software is designed for policymaking, hence its functions must be relevant in this context and the relevance must be clearly conveyed either through short explanations or longer tutorials. A consequence is to avoid the temptation to implement functions just because we can, as may happen during software development cycles that gradually lose track of their intended audience. For instance, while network science has proposed many measures, the 'Measure' button provides access to few measures but emphasizes their meaning in a policy context. Similarly, two policy maps can be compared on many possible features, but the 'Compare' button contrasts two policy networks based on features such as the presence and types of feedback loops.

3.3   Implementation of the Five Functionalities

A video demonstration of the five functionalities in `ActionableSystems` is provided at https://youtu.be/OdKJW8tNDcM. The first three key functionalities are accessed via the top panel (Fig. 4), after clicking on the 'See' button. The analysis of cycles (functionality 1) gives access to a list of all cycles, and each one is displayed by arranging the content as a circle (Fig. 5a). When finding paths (functionality 2), we use a pop-up window whose design implements recommendations from our previous usability study [23]. Users select the end and start node, either through a drop-down menu or by typing a few letters and using auto-complete. End-nodes that are greyed out cannot be reached from the selected starting node, whereas black end-nodes can be reached from at least one path. When one or more paths exist, they are graphically organized so the user can see the different paths (Fig. 5c). To find rippling effects (functionality 3), users choose the factor on which to intervene, and how far

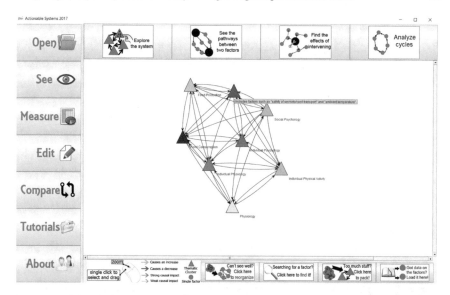

Fig. 4 Rendering the System Dynamics model from Verigin et al. [18] in `ActionableSystems` with a hierarchical visualization. Each policy domain is shown as a thematic cluster (triangle). Hovering over a cluster shows examples of its content, while clicking on it will unpack the factors that it contains. Tools to find rippling effects, paths, and cycles are at the top

they want to be screening for rippling effects. The result is organized in concentric circles to emphasize 'rippling' effects (Fig. 5b). Participants can import definitions and evidence *en masse* via the 'data' button (Fig. 4, bottom right). The evidence can be viewed, edited or created (functionality 4) by clicking on a factor and opening an editor within a pop-up window.

While previous software opened files created by 'similar' software (Table 1), our software works across domains. Specifically, it opens maps created by visualization, argumentation, and simulation tools (functionality 5). To connect with network visualization software (e.g., `Gephi` and `Visone`), we use the GraphML format which is defined as a common (XML-based) format for exchanging graph data in a visualization context [35]. We connect with argumentation software (`Cmap` and `Coggle`) by reading files in their own formats, and similarly we access data from simulation software such as `MentalModeler` by reading its own format. As the idea of integrating in a workflow means that we can get data both in *and out*, all results generated by users can be saved. For instance, the whole list of cycles can be exported with the "Save cycles" button (Fig. 5 bottom), and the same applies to pathways, or results obtained via the 'Measure' or 'Edit' button.

Finally, maps being *representations* of systems, they may depart from the real system depending on how they were created. Understanding these discrepancies is important when policymakers base their analysis off maps. `ActionableSystems` provides a summary of a map: in Fig. 6, we see that the Foresight Map has a roughly

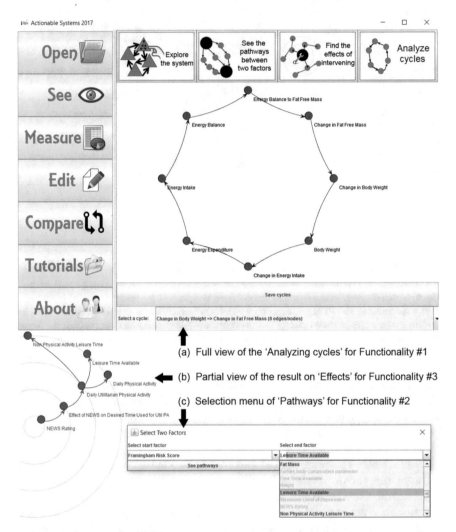

Fig. 5 Key functionalities for the System Dynamics model from Verigin et al. [18]: **a** a cycle with 8 nodes, **b** rippling effects of intervening on the NEWS rating up to depth 3, and **c** searching for paths starting at the Framingham Risk Score

equal share of reinforcing and balancing loops. Our software also allows to contrast two maps: for instance, a second map designed for the same context differs significantly as it almost exclusively involves reinforcing loops. Such differences can be important for policymakers, as one map may show few balancing loops about a problem, thus suggesting that the problem is much less controllable than shown in another map.

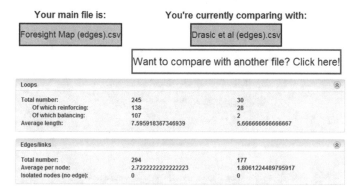

Fig. 6 Comparison of the Foresight Map (left) with the PHSA obesity and well-being map [15], using metrics such as the number and types of loops

4 Demonstrations

4.1 Public Health Policy on Obesity and Well-Being

In 2013, the Provincial Health Services Authority of British Columbia authored a discussion paper on the inter-relationships among obesity, overweight, weight bias and mental well-being [36]. The paper narrated the evidence, but did not visually represent it. As a follow-up, we created a map of obesity and well-being [15]. Using ActionableSystems, we can now ask key policy questions from the map.

First, we can investigate in which ways weight bias affects mental well-being, in the context of obesity. This is an essential question, whose answers runs through the pages of the previous discussion paper but were not previously available in a simple, synthesized form. Using the tool for disjoint paths in ActionableSystems, we immediately know that there are 6 disjoint paths (Fig. 7a). They vary in length from a direct impact of weight bias on mental well-being (length 1) to a path going towards depression and its effect on physical health (length 5). The PHSA map is annotated, as its causal connections have a strength and a type (either a causal increase or decrease). This information allows us to more precisely understand the type of paths running from weight stigma to mental well-being. The composition rule for causal effects (often used in System Dynamics) can intuitively be understood as a multiplication: if A increases ($\times 1$) B, and B decreases C ($\times - 1$), then A decreases C ($1 \times -1 = -1$). More formally, in a causal path, an odd number of causal decreases leads to the path representing an overall decrease. In Fig. 7a, we observe that all of the paths have an odd number of red edges (i.e. causal decrease), that is, weight bias decreases mental well-being in six different ways. One practical implication is as follows. Assuming that we cannot completely eliminate weight bias, we try to limit its consequences. Making improvements along well-known paths (e.g., unhealthy weight control practices, lack of access to health professionals) may not be sufficient

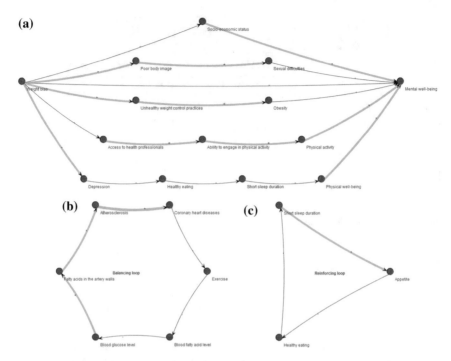

Fig. 7 Visualizations of the PHSA obesity and well-being map [15] showing pathways from weight stigma to mental well-being (**a**), and two examples of balancing loops (**b–c**)

to counter-act the challenges that individuals experience through other paths. This view thus promotes a more holistic approach to policymaking.

Second, identifying potential policy levers requires a deep understanding of what already drives the dynamics of the system. Loops are important drivers, either to balance (odd number of causal decreases) or to amplify dynamics. Finegood has long suggested that "new methods are likely required to assist stakeholders in [...] creating new feedback loops as a means to shifting the dominance away from [the loops that] currently give rise to obesity" [37]. ActionableSystems provides support in this regard, by allowing policymakers to list all loops and their types. Figure 7b shows a balancing loop, where heart diseases reduce exercises, which in turn increases the likeliness for heart diseases. Policymakers need to counter-act this undesirable loop, but cannot simply 'remove' it because most of it involves physiological causes (which are outside their control). They can thus add to the system by supporting exercise-based cardiac rehabilitation, which has been proven to reduce cardiovascular mortality in an updated 2016 Cochrane systematic review [38]. This will 'take away' from the balancing loop and promote exercise. Conversely, Fig. 7c shows a reinforcing loop in which individuals eat less healthily. The 'Tragedy of the Commons' in System Dynamics suggests that, if a harmful loop needs a resource and this resource cannot be directly modified, then a less harmful loop could be created in order to tap into that same resource and deplete it. Rather than telling individuals to just eat less, an approach can be to promote the consumption of healthy foods (e.g., high in fibers) which should deplete 'appetite' as the resource and consequently have individuals eat less unhealthy foods. While seeing disjoint paths clearly shows policymakers what should be monitored for an intervention, training is needed to translate loops into practical policy actions. For instance, identifying a harmful loop and thinking of making another harmful loop to counter-act it would not be straight-forwardly inferred from the picture, but instead requires expertise in the field and some familiarity with systems thinking.

4.2 Public Health Nutrition

Public health nutrition aims at improving the nutritional profile of the population (e.g., not deriving too much energy from fat or sugar, not exceeding a given sodium consumption), which will improve population health. Computational methods were recently used to assess the populations current profile [39], and our software complement such methods to find and evaluate interventions. Consider that a policymaker wants an intervention that improves healthy eating, and needs to evaluate the health effects as changes in disease burden measured in quality-adjusted life-year (QALY). The policymaker has access to a broad range of existing models which can turn various physiological measures into QALY. The process thus consists of (i) identifying what physiological changes are triggered by a nutrition campaign, (ii) selecting the changes that can be used as input to available models, and (iii) connecting these inputs using the new layer.

Without ActionableSystems, the first step may consist of navigating the parts of a large map devoted to nutrition and physiology (Fig. 8a). Instead, with our software, the policymaker can anchor the system in healthy eating, and ask to see what gets affected up to a given distance (Fig. 8b). The policymaker would then visually scan the factors, and note that 'blood pressure' is affected. Since the policymaker has models on how changes in blood pressure translates to QALY, blood pressure is selected as the desired model input. For the new policy layer, the policymaker needs to identify the various ways in which the policy (improving healthy eating) affects the models input (blood pressure). Using our software, the disjoint path tool is sufficient to generate such layer, and provides the five different paths linking the healthy eating to blood pressure.

5 Discussion and Conclusion

We designed a new software solution to support policymakers in navigating complex systems, and demonstrated its possibilities in obesity research and public health nutrition. Our software integrates with visualization, argumentation, and simulation

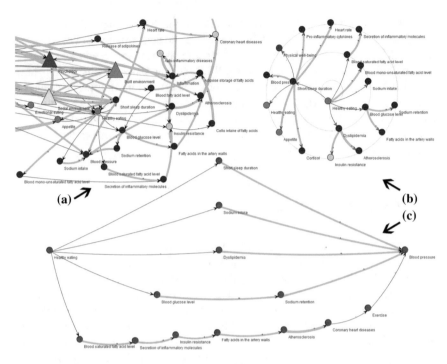

Fig. 8 Visualization of a large map (**a**), followed by identification of possible consequences of healthy eating (**b**), and multiple paths for one selected consequence (**c**)

tools. However, there are several other types of important tools in policymaking [27]. As we explained, integrating with such tools is important to make the best use of existing data. Several integrations are particularly interesting avenues for future work.

Integrating with opinion mining tools can be particularly useful for public health informatics. Indeed, policymakers need to know what constituents support in a policy [40]. If this was readily accessible as a map, they would be able to more easily find policies that can positively impact the dynamics of the system *and* are endorsed by constituents. This integration would not significantly alter the design of our software (e.g., the level of endorsement can be visually shown through edge patterns).

Similarly, integrating with tools for ontologies would only expand the list of file formats that can be opened, and would not change the software beyond this (since the ontology would be displayed as a network). This integration would enable policymakers to access the many systems which are represented as ontologies. For instance, it would give access to the One Health Ontology (OHO), a network of ontologies including human heath, used in other chapters of this book.

Other types of integration may call for new designs. In particular, eParticipation tools require an online, distributed design. In contrast, our software and all the other solutions reviewed are designed for a single user. The next frontier in public health informatics is to develop tools that allow multiple users to navigate complex systems, and possibly in an asynchronous manner (i.e. when not all users are interacting with the software at the same time). This will require new designs and usability studies, but the effort also comes with the promise of a more inclusive approach to policy-making and a more comprehensive exploration of complex systems.

Acknowledgements Research reported in this publication was supported by the Global Obesity Prevention Center (GOPC) at Johns Hopkins, and the Eunice Kennedy Shriver National Institute of Child Health and Human Development (NICHD) and the Office of The Director, National Institutes of Health (OD) under award number U54HD070725. The content is solely the responsibility of authors and does not necessarily represent the official views of the National Institute of Health.

Appendix: Glossary

- **Layer**: expansion of a policy-oriented simulation model to capture the relationships between the models input. These relationships are represented in the form of a network.
- **Map**: a representation of an existing system in the form of a network.
- **Model**: a simplification of a system, model or phenomena in a computerized form.
- **Policy**: a set of interventions proposed or implemented by local authorities, government, business, or individuals.

References

1. Galea S, Roux AVD, Simon CP, Kaplan GA (2017) Using complex systems approaches in the study of population health and health disparities: seven observations, pp 297–304
2. Zhang D, Giabbanelli PJ, Arah O, Zimmerman F (2014) Am J Public Health 104(7):1217
3. Giabbanelli PJ, Alimadad A, Dabbaghian V, Finegood DT (2012) J Comput Sci 3(1):17
4. Giabbanelli PJ et al (2014) Modelling the joint effect of social determinants and peers on obesity among canadian adults, pp 145–160
5. Preventive Medicine (2013) 57(5):434
6. Bahr D, Browning R, Wyatt H, Hill J (2009) Obesity 17(4):723
7. Homer J, Milstein B, Dietz W, Buchner D, Majestic E (2006) In: 24th International system dynamics conference
8. Levy D et al (2010) Obesity Rev 12:378
9. Shoham D, Hammond R, Rahmandad H, Wang Y, Hovmand P (2015) Curr Epidemiol Rep 2:71
10. Rivis A, Sheeran P (2002) Curr Psychol 22(2):218
11. Stok F, Ridder D, Vet E, Wit J (2014) Br J Health Psychol 19(1):52
12. Jain R (1990) The art of computer systems performance analysis: techniques for experimental design, measurement, simulation, and modeling. Wiley
13. Giabbanelli PJ, Crutzen R (2017) Comput Math Methods Med 2017:5742629
14. Vandenbroeck I, Goossens J, Clemens M (2007) Government Office for Science, UK Governments Foresight Programme
15. Drasic L, Giabbanelli P (2015) Can J Diabetes 39:S12

16. Giabbanelli PJ, Tornsney-Weir T, Mago VK (2012) Appl Soft Syst 12:3711
17. Giles B et al (2007) Soc Sci Med 64(3):562
18. Verigin T, Giabbanelli PJ, Davidsen PI (2016) In: Proceedings of the 49th annual simulation symposium, (ANSS-16). pp 9:1–9:10
19. Struben J, Chan D, Dube L (2014) N Y Acad Sci Ann 1331:57
20. Voinov A, Shugart HH (2013) Environ Model Softw 39:149
21. Knapen R, Janssen S, Roosenschoon O, Verweij P, de Winter W, Uiterwijk M, Wien JE (2013) Environ Model Softw 39:274
22. Giabbanelli PJ, Gray SA, Aminpour P (2017) Environ Model Softw 95:320
23. Giabbanelli P, Flarsheim R, Vesuvala C, Drasic L (2016) Obes Rev 17:194
24. Hall KD et al (2011) Lancet 378(9793):826
25. Siokou C, Morgan R, Shiell A (2014) Public Health Res Pract 25(1)
26. Dorner D (1996) The logic of failure: recognizing and avoiding error in complex situations. Addison-Wesley, Reading, Massachusetts
27. Kamateri E et al (2015) A comparative analysis of tools and technologies for policy making. Springer International Publishing, pp 125–156
28. Skyttner L (2006) General systems theory. World Scientific
29. Hamid TK (2009) Thinking in circles about obesity, 2nd edn. Springer
30. Ross S (1974) Structure of decision: the cognitive maps of political elites. In: Complexity and the presidency: gouverneur Morris in the constitutional convention. Princeton University Press, pp 96–112
31. Axelrod R (1974) Structure of decision: the cognitive maps of political elites. In: Results. Princeton University Press, pp 221–250
32. Vennix JA (1996) Group model building. In: Individual and organizational problem construction. Wiley, pp 9–41
33. Congdon KG, Congdon DC (1986) Vis Arts Res 12(12):73
34. Dustin DL, Bricker KS, Schwab KA (2009) Leis Sci 32(1):3
35. Brandes U, Eiglsperger M, Lerner J, Pich C (2013) Graph markup language (GraphML)
36. Provincial Health Services Authority of British Columbia. From weight to well-being: Time for a shift in paradigms? (2013). http://www.phsa.ca/population-public-health-site/Documents/W2WBTechnicalReport_20130208FINAL.pdf
37. Finegood D (2011) The oxford handbook of the social science of obesity. In: The complex systems science of obesity, pp 208–236
38. Anderson L et al (2016) J Am Coll Cardiol 67(1):1
39. Giabbanelli PJ, Adams J (2016) Public Health Nutr 19(9):1543–1551
40. Giabbanelli PJ, Adams J, Pillutla VS (2016) Feasibility and framing of interventions based on public support: leveraging text analytics for policymakers. Springer, pp 188–200

Part II
Modeling and Simulation

An Agent-Based Model of Healthy Eating with Applications to Hypertension

Amin Khademi, Donglan Zhang, Philippe J. Giabbanelli, Shirley Timmons, Chengqian Luo and Lu Shi

Abstract Changing descriptive social norm in health behavior ("how many people are behaving healthy") has been shown to be effective in promoting healthy eating. We developed an agent-based model to explore the potential of changing social norm in reducing hypertension among the adult population of Los Angeles County. The model uses the 2007 California Health Interview Survey (CHIS) to create a virtual population that mimics the joint distribution of demographic characteristics and health behavior in the Los Angeles County. We calibrated the outcome of hypertension as a function of individual age and fruits/vegetable consumption, based upon the observed pattern in the survey. We then simulated an intervention scenario to promote healthier eating by increasing the visibility (i.e. descriptive social norms) of those who eat at least one serving of fruits/vegetable per day. We compare the hypertension incidence under the status quo scenario and the intervention scenario. We found that the effect size of 5% in social norm enhancement yields a reduction in 5 year hypertension incidence by 10.08%. An effect size of 15% would reduce incidence by 15.50%. In conclusion, the agent-based model built and calibrated around real-world data shows that changes descriptive social norms in healthy eating can be effective to reduce the burden of hypertension. The model can be improved in

A. Khademi · C. Luo
Department of Industrial Engineering, Clemson University, Clemson, SC 29634, USA
e-mail: khademi@clemson.edu

D. Zhang
Department of Health Policy and Management, University of Georgia, Athens,
GA 30602, USA
e-mail: dzhang@uga.edu

P. J. Giabbanelli (✉)
Computer Science Department, Furman University, Greenville, SC 29613, USA
e-mail: giabbanelli@gmail.com

S. Timmons
School of Nursing, Clemson University, Clemson, SC 29634, USA
e-mail: stimmon@clemson.edu

L. Shi
Department of Public Health Sciences, Clemson University, Clemson, SC 29634, USA
e-mail: lus@clemson.edu

© Springer International Publishing AG, part of Springer Nature 2018   43
P. J. Giabbanelli et al. (eds.), *Advanced Data Analytics in Health*, Smart Innovation,
Systems and Technologies 93, https://doi.org/10.1007/978-3-319-77911-9_3

the future by also including the chronic conditions that are affected by changes in fruits/vegetable consumption.

1 Introduction

Models can serve many different goals [1], some of which do not require any data. For example, models can test the implications or robustness of theories, and the process of developing a model can guide future data collection efforts. However, data is essential for many models, and particularly in the context of health policy. Data can be used for calibration and validation both by explanatory models (whose goal may be to establish which theory best replicates existing data) or by predictive models (whose baseline can be grounded in existing data). Modeling and simulation (M&S) is now one of the many tools used in public health, where it also appears under the umbrella of 'systems science' [2, 3]. A particular benefit of M&S is the ability to provide a virtual laboratory, in which policy scenarios (also called 'what-if questions' more generally) can be safely tested [4]. Its application within public health spans a broad spectrum from infectious diseases [5] to chronic conditions [6, 7] such as smoking [8] and obesity [9]. Eating behaviors have received particular attention in modeling studies, either as one of the drivers of weight-related factors within studies on obesity [10, 11], or as the main object of study [12, 13]. In this chapter, we develop an Agent-Based Model (ABM) for eating behaviors. It is a predictive model (also known as 'prospective') rather than a descriptive model (also known as 'retrospective'): it seeks to simulate what may happen in the future. Data is essential for the quality of this model, both to capture the key features and behaviors in the population, and to ensure that the model aligns with real-world data before using it to simulate virtual interventions.

Many M&S techniques can be used for a specific problem such as eating behaviors. Other techniques such as Fuzzy Cognitive Maps are illustrated through the chapters of this book. ABM is a discrete, individual-oriented technique. That is, each entity is explicitly represented. In the case of eating behaviors, the entities would be the individuals from the target population. In addition, entities interact with each other and/or their environment through discrete time steps. These aspects are important ones to capture when modeling eating behavior, given the heterogeneity [14] among members of the population (which can be accounted for by representing each member), and the fact that behavior changes as a result of socio-environmental interactions [15]. In our model, we particularly seek to capture social norms on healthy eating (for possible policy intervention) and the prevalence of hypertension (as the measured policy outcome). Social norms change through social ties, represented by interactions between agents. Changes in social norms may then impact eating behaviors, which can ultimately change the prevalence of hypertension.

Section 2 provides background information on changing social norms as particular type of public health intervention, and on the potential for addressing hypertension through social norms around food choices. Section 3 details the development of the ABM, and highlights its dependence on data. In Sect. 4, we use the model to investigate policy interventions of different strengths. Finally, we discuss how the model can still be improved, and the implications of our findings for public health.

The main contributions of this chapter are twofold:
- We demonstrate the development of an Agent-Based Model for predictive analytics in health.
- We use the model to examine interventions for hypertension.

2 Background

A major determinant of human eating behavior is "social norm," a mechanism whereby people model what and how much to eat after others' eating behavior [16]. A wealth of experimental studies and commentaries has demonstrated the effect of social influence on eating, dating back to the 1980s [17]. Social norms can be injunctive (i.e. beliefs about what others approve of) or descriptive (i.e. expectation of others' pattern of behavior). Studies in behavioral science have suggested that enhancing descriptive rather than injunctive norm messages can effectively improve peoples adherence to healthy behaviors [18, 19]. This evidence, consistently observed from cross-sectional studies, experimental studies and meta-analysis [18, 19], offers an opportunity to increase the effectiveness of population health interventions. That is, an individual who successfully changes his/her health behavior may simultaneously improve the social norm influencing the other interconnected individuals' behavior. As a result, there is growing interest in developing effective interventions to change social norms in healthy eating [20].

Fresh fruit and vegetable intake is associated with a lower risk of developing hypertension [21], a prevalent, costly and preventable chronic condition that leads to many morbidity and mortality outcomes [22]. Among various prevention programs aiming at controlling hypertension, improving consumption of fruits and vegetables is a potentially effective lifestyle modification that could reduce high blood pressure both in people with hypertension and in those at risk for developing hypertension within a relatively short time period [23]. However, promoting fruit and vegetable intake is not easy. As was shown in the Behavioral Risk Factor Surveillance System, the percentage of U.S. adults who consumed fruit (60.8%) or vegetable (77.1%) one or more times per day continued to remain unchanged, whereas nutrition scientists have recommended eating five or more servings of fruits and vegetables on a daily basis [24].

The prevalence of high blood pressure among adults in Los Angeles County (LAC) saw relatively small change from 2004 to 2014 (24–25.8%) [25]. In the present study, we intend to simulate a norm-changing intervention that promotes fruit and vegetable intake to explore the degree to which it could reduce the burden of hypertension in LAC. Based on the design and evidence from two randomized control trials [19], the hypothetical intervention used a media campaign to send the true information such that "above 90% of people in your community are eating fruit and vegetables daily", to enhance the influence of individuals who have a healthier diet within their social networks [12, 26], therefore reciprocally highlights the descriptive social norm of healthy eating.

This reciprocal behavioral mechanism has not been extensively studied as many studies assumed that individuals behave independently [12]. To explore the potential of this norm-changing intervention requires the simulation of the interaction process between individuals, a mechanism that can be best captured by agent-based modeling (ABM) [27]. Based upon our previous validated model for healthy eating [12, 28, 29] we build an agent-based model of hypertension as an outcome of fruit and vegetable consumption in this study. Simulations were performed to examine the effect of an intervention containing messages of descriptive social norms for healthy eating on control of hypertension prevalence in a 5 year time period.

3   Development of the Agent-Based Model (ABM)

3.1   Overview

Our ABM captures how individuals consume fruit and vegetable based on (i) their initial preferences, (ii) social norms, and (iii) individual characteristics such as age and gender. This part of the model was previously published in [12] for a health-audience, thus we will describe it briefly here and emphasize the modeling aspects. We then link fruit and vegetable consumption as well as individual characteristics to the risk for hypertension. This 'extension' to the initial model allows to establish how a virtual intervention affects hypertension. A virtual intervention cannot change (i) one's *initial* preferences since that cannot be immediately altered, or (iii) characteristics such as age or gender whose dynamics are outside the control of a health policy. Consequently, the intervention can only target (ii) social norms. Nevertheless, it is important to represent (i) and (iii) in the model as they also affect the prevalence of hypertension, which is the target for the intervention. The following sub-sections detail the previously developed core of the model for fruit and vegetable consumption, then explain its extension for the study of hypertension. Our model is implemented in Java. It is open source and publicly accessible on a third-party repository.[1] This section ends by specifying the whole ABM using the updated ODD (Overview, Design concepts, and Details) protocol, which is the standard for describing an ABM at a high level [30].

---

[1]https://osf.io/m3w9g/.

3.2 Core ABM: Modeling Fruit and Vegetable Consumption

3.2.1 Individual Preferences

Individuals have preferences regarding the Taste T (the stronger the preference, the more the individual prefers sweet and salty food) and Healthfulness H of food (the stronger, the more the individual cares about the healthiness of food). We use the Food Attitudes and Behavior (FAB) Survey [31] from 2007, which comprised 3,397 adults and aimed to evaluate various factors such as attitudes and beliefs that are related to eating behaviors among adults. We applied a probit regression, which employs a probit link function to estimate the parameters for taste preference and preference for healthy foods. The regression takes the following form, where Pr denotes probability: $Pr(Y = 1|X) = \Phi(X'B)$. Taste preference is related to age by:

$$\left\{ \begin{array}{c} \text{if } age \in [18\text{--}54], \text{ then } T \text{ is uniformly drawn from } [0.25, 1] \\ \text{if } age \in [55+], \text{ then } T \text{ is uniformly drawn from } [0, 0.75] \end{array} \right\} \tag{1}$$

Preferences for healthy foods are also drawn uniformly at random based on age, gender, and (denoted by $\wedge$) educational attainment ('HS' denotes high school):

$$\left\{ \begin{array}{c} \text{if } age \in [18\text{--}54] \wedge gender = male, \text{ then } H \in [0, 0.75] \\ \text{if } age \in [55+] \wedge gender = male \wedge education < HS, \text{ then } H \in [0, 0.75] \\ \text{if } age \in [18\text{--}54] \wedge gender = female \wedge education < HS, \text{ then } H \in [0, 0.75] \\ \text{otherwise } H \in [0.25, 1] \end{array} \right\} \tag{2}$$

The parameterization underlying Eqs. 1 and 2 is as follows. In the FAB survey, taste preference was measured on a 5-point likert scale as "I like sweet foods" and "I like salty foods" in the FAB survey. The preference for healthy foods is also measured on a 5-point likert scale as "I have a strong value for eating healthy". We rescaled these preferences to be bounded between 0 and 1 (where 1 indicates stronger preferences) using the formula $\frac{X - Min}{Max}$ where X is the original variable, for which Min and Max compute the minimum and maximum values respectively. The average preferences are above 0.5, indicating that the respondents in the FAB survey have relatively strong taste and health value. We then estimated the relationship between individual characteristics and the preferences using ordered logit regression models. Probit and logit models are among the most commonly used methods to estimate probabilities for categories [32]. The preference for one method or another depends on fields, where public health researchers prefer logit because it produces odds ratio while economists often use probit regressions because it estimates marginal effects directly. The coefficients are usually undifferentiated. In the regression, preferences were used as dependent variables and individual characteristics as independent variables. As shown in Eqs. 1 and 2, age, being female and educational attainment are positively associated with preferences for healthy foods, while age is negatively associated with taste preference. We predicted the range of values for preferences across age groups (18–34, 35–54, 55 and above), gender (male or female) and educational attainment. For example, preferences were predicted as if every person was 18–34 year old, controlling for all other person-level characteristics in the regression model; it was then predicted again assuming everyone to be 35–54 years old, and so on. The ranges for the values under those scenarios were summarized and represented in Eqs. 1 and 2.

3.2.2 Social Norms

Preferences may change due to shifts in social norms. As discussed in the background, social norms around foods mean that what and how much an individual eats also depends on the eating behavior of peers [16]. Modeling social norms thus leads to modeling how individuals interact, which is one of the strengths of using ABM. In a model, interactions between individuals can be divided in two parts: *who* individuals interact with, and *how*? Simulations of social networks commonly account for the small-world property which states that (i) individuals belong to groups, and (ii) there are ties between groups such as an individual is on average only a few ties away from any other. Consequently, social ties between our agents are a (static) small-world network. While the Watts-Strogatz (WS) model is a typical network generator to obtain the small-world property, it does so using randomness, which in turns introduces more randomness in the ABM as a whole and thus calls for more runs of a simulation. Research in graph theory has shown that small-world networks could be created without randomness while having parameters to precisely control them (e.g. in terms of network size and degree) [33]. We thus use a deterministic variation of the WS model [11]. The component of our simulation in charge of generating networks has been validated through several studies [34, 35].

In accordance to the multi-level theory of population health, an individual's preferences change in response to the preferences of friends in the social network, while retaining their own 'habits' to a certain degree [36]. Here habits represent an individual's own taste preference and preference for healthy foods, which originate from their historic exposures and experiences. Formally, preferences in taste and healthfulness for an individual i at time t are denoted by $T_{i,t}$ and $H_{i,t}$ respectively. The balance between one's own habits and the importance of peers' norms is denoted by $\alpha_i \in (0, 0.3]$, where larger values represent greater susceptibility to influence from friends. This range was chosen in a previous study [12] to represent that peers may be an important driver for one's habits, but they are not the only driver and cannot alter most of one's behavior within a single time step. Susceptibility varies between individuals, thus the value of α depends on the individual i and it is initially drawn from a uniform probability distribution. In the absence of any marketing strategy to promote either healthy or unhealthy norms, each friend carries an equal influence and thus an individual's taste preferences and health beliefs represent the balance between the average habits of friends and her own at $t - 1$. Therefore, the following two equations provide the taste preferences and health beliefs in the absence of exogenous influences on social norms [12]:

$$T_{i,t} = (1 - \alpha_i) \times T_{i,t-1} + \alpha_i \times \frac{\sum_{j \in friends(i)} T_{j,t-1}}{\sum_{j \in friends(i)} 1} \tag{3}$$

$$H_{i,t} = (1 - \alpha_i) \times H_{i,t-1} + \alpha_i \times \frac{\sum_{j \in friends(i)} H_{j,t-1}}{\sum_{j \in friends(i)} 1} \tag{4}$$

In these two equations, note that $\sum_{j \in friends(i)} 1$ is simply the number of friends for agent i, hence the denominator may be re-written if one introduced a specified notation such as $d(i)$ for the degree of i.

In the presence of the exogenous influence of social media, an individual term $\gamma \in (-1, 1)$ is introduced. In other words, γ represents the influence of the media campaign (if any) on an individual's perception of social norm in the person's social network. A positive γ represents advertisements for unhealthy foods, which has two effects. First, it *emphasizes* taste preferences. That is, peers with stronger taste preferences have more visibility as they better fit the norm that is promoted ($1 + \gamma$ multiplicative weight when $T_{j,t-1} > T_{i,t-1}$), while peers with lower taste preferences are less visible ($1 - \gamma$ multiplicative weight when $T_{j,t-1} < T_{i,t-1}$). Second, it lowers the importance of healthy foods (e.g., the advertisements show the enjoyment of eating foods which may have high-sugar high-fat content). In a symmetric way to taste preferences, peers who value healthy foods carry less impact ($1 - \gamma$ multiplicative weight when $H_{j,t-1} > H_{i,t-1}$) while those who echo the promoted norm have more impact ($1 + \gamma$ multiplicative weight when $H_{j,t-1} < H_{i,t-1}$). Consequently, the social norm component of each preference can be seen as being made of two parts, to increase and decrease the strength of peer influences relatively to one's own preferences. Note that when γ is negative, we promote healthy foods, and its multiplicative effect is the opposite of promoting unhealthy foods as described. The preferences of an individual are thus updated using the following equations:

$$T_{i,t} = (1 - \alpha_i) \times T_{i,t-1} + \alpha_i \times \frac{\sum_{\substack{j \in friends(i) \\ T_{j,t-1} > T_{i,t-1}}} (1+\gamma) \times T_{j,t-1} + \sum_{\substack{j \in friends(i) \\ T_{j,t-1} \leq T_{i,t-1}}} (1-\gamma) \times T_{j,t-1}}{\sum_{\substack{j \in friends(i) \\ T_{j,t-1} > T_{i,t-1}}} (1+\gamma) + \sum_{\substack{j \in friends(i) \\ T_{j,t-1} \leq T_{i,t-1}}} (1-\gamma)} \tag{5}$$

$$H_{i,t} = (1 - \alpha_i) \times H_{i,t-1} + \alpha_i \times \frac{\sum_{\substack{j \in friends(i) \\ H_{j,t-1} > H_{i,t-1}}} (1-\gamma) \times H_{j,t-1} + \sum_{\substack{j \in friends(i) \\ H_{j,t-1} \leq H_{i,t-1}}} (1+\gamma) \times H_{j,t-1}}{\sum_{\substack{j \in friends(i) \\ H_{j,t-1} > H_{i,t-1}}} (1-\gamma) + \sum_{\substack{j \in friends(i) \\ H_{j,t-1} \leq H_{i,t-1}}} (1+\gamma)} \tag{6}$$

3.2.3 Demographic Variables

The demographic variables for the population of our ABM consist of the age category (18–34, 35–54, and over 55), the gender (male or female), and educational

Table 1 Demographic variables based on a subsample of the CHIS 2007 [37]

Demographic variables	Category	Percentage (%)
Gender	Male	39.29
	Female	60.71
Age group (years)	18–34	28.64
	35–64	39.59
	65+	31.77
Educational attainment	Less than high school	12.33
	High school	30.45
	Some college	30.00
	College	27.22

attainment (less than high school, high school, some college, or college). The value of these three variables are set randomly and independently for each agent in line with the proportions for the target population (Table 1) reported in the Los Angeles County subsample of the California Health Interview Survey (CHIS) 2007 (survey weights adjusted) [37]. The number of agents in the simulation is not limited by the equations and distributions of our model, thus it would at first seem trivial to set up a virtual population matching the whole of Los Angeles County (9,818,605 individuals per the 2010 United State Census). However, there are two limitations on the population size of an ABM. First, there are implementation and hardware limits. Simulating more individuals may require more memory and more computations, which could be solved using high-performance computing (HPC) clusters or cloud computing. Second, a more subtle point is that the ability to create an arbitrary number n of agents assumes that all components of the model can set up these n agents. This may not be true, particularly for the component in charge of generating social interactions between agents (i.e. the network generator). Indeed, network generators are not all able to create any network of size n because their smallest unit may not be one agent but a set of agents [38]. For example, hierarchical network models create and repeatedly copy groups of agents, thus their smallest unit is a group and not a single agent (e.g. they could generate a network of size $4 \times 5 = 20$ or $4 \times 6 = 24$ but not 21, 22, or 23). Due to limitations in both the implementation and the network generator, our population has 10,000 agents.

3.2.4 Probability to Eat Fruit and Vegetable

We finally estimated the probability to eat fruit and vegetable (FV) given the model components detailed above. Since the population's daily serving of fruit and vegetable is mostly less than 5 but greater than 1, eating two servings or less of FV was taken as the division between sufficient and insufficient consumption of FV [39]. Thus, the daily probability of consuming fruit and vegetable is the probability of consuming at least 2 servings of FV a day. This probability was estimated using a probit regression (as was employed for preferences). We used the coefficients βs, estimated using the standard maximum likelihood from the regression, as parameters for the FV equation. For variables that were not measured in the FAB data, we obtained coefficients (aka priors) from other empirical studies (described below), and subtracted a fixed effect from the constant. The probability of eating at least two servings of fruit and vegetables per day is given by:

$$Pr(FV > 1)_{i,t} = \beta_0 + \beta_1 \times T_{i,t} + \beta_2 \times H_{i,t} + \beta_3 \times PS_i \times PI_{fv} + \beta_4 \times PS_i \times PI_{ff}$$
$$+ \beta_5 \times A_{FV,i,t} + \beta_6 \times age_i + \beta_0 \times gender_i + \beta_8 \times education_i$$
(7)

The formula above bounds the outcome in the range 0–1.

Our **empirical measurement** puts items from the FAB survey in relation with variables of the equation in the following way. The price sensitivity PS_i was measured by "I don't eat fruit and vegetables as much as I like because they cost too much", and food accessibility $A_{FV,i,t}$ was defined as "It is hard for me to purchase fruit and vegetables in my neighborhood" and "When I eat out, it is easy for me to get fruit and vegetables". The questions are chosen in the survey based on associated references that have demonstrated good reliability [31]. The FAB survey also queries the age, gender, educational attainment and race/ethnicity of the respondents. It should be noted that income is not measured in the FAB survey; accordingly, educational attainment is used instead of income as a proxy measure for socioeconomic status in the model. This may be a reasonable approximation since educational attainment is related to income [40].

Coefficients on price indices (both PI_{fv} for FV and their counterpart of 'unhealthy' fast-foods PI_{ff}) were obtained from [41] and [42], which estimated how FV consumption probabilities was impacted by the fruit and vegetables price index and the fast food price index. All coefficient values are summarized in Table 2.

3.3 Extension: Modeling Hypertension

At the beginning of the first year in the simulation, each individual's hypertension status is randomly assigned according to the prevalence data in different age groups from the CHIS. In CHIS, hypertension status was measured by self-reported "ever diagnosed as having hypertension" and/or currently taking anti-hypertensive medications. The probabilities for having hypertension at baseline were: 7% for those aged 18–34, 20.9% for those aged 35–54, and 52.9% for those aged over 55. An individual *without* hypertension at the beginning of a year has a probability $Pr(Hypertension)_{i,Y_0}$ of developing hypertension at the *end* of this first year depending on the fruit and vegetable intake, specified by Eq. 7. The risk equation that calculates the effect of fruit and vegetable consumption on hypertension status is estimated from the CHIS datasets using logistic regression. Since CHIS is a repeated cross-sectional survey, from which we are not able to get data on hypertension

Table 2 Coefficients in Eq. 7

Coefficient	Value	Data source
β_0	−0.3	FAB survey
β_1	−0.3	FAB survey
β_2	1.0	FAB survey
β_3	−0.2	FAB survey and [41]
β_4	0.1	FAB survey and [41]
β_5	0.2	FAB survey
β_6	0 if $age_i \in [18, 34]$, 0.1 if $age_i \in [35 - 54]$, 0.2 if $age_i \geq 55$	FAB survey
β_7	0 if $gender_i = male$, 0.1 if $gender_i = female$	FAB survey
β_8	0 if $education_i <$ high school, 0.1 if $education_i =$ high school, 0.3 otherwise	FAB survey

incidence directly, the parameters in the risk equation are then calibrated to fit for the population-weighted trend of hypertension prevalence in LAC from 2007 to 2012. The calibration criterion is that the simulated hypertension prevalence should be within the 95% confidence interval of the observed hypertension prevalence estimated from the 2012 CHIS data. The probability of having hypertension at the end of the first year is:

$$Pr(Hypertension)_{i,Y_0} = MAX(0.0, 0.002 - 0.000055 \times age^2 + 0.01 \times age + log(0.69) \times \frac{\text{number of days eating fruit and vegetables in a year}}{365} \qquad (8)$$

The number of days for which a person has eaten more than one serving of fruit and/or vegetable is calculated by applying $Pr(FV > 1)_{i,t}$ each day of the year (per Eq. 7). The *max* function ensures that the model-generated probability of having hypertension is non-negative. We note that the quadratic curve has a positive coefficient of age and a negative coefficient of age squared, which echoes the pattern of diminishing marginal impact of age on hypertension [43].

Individuals who have not been diagnosed with hypertension at baseline or by the end of the first year may still develop it in the subsequent years. From the end of year 2 onward, we use the following equation calibrated on the 2007–2012 CHIS data:

$$Pr(Hypertension)_{i,Y_n} = MAX(0.0, 0.002 - 0.000055 \times age^2 + 0.01 \times age + log(0.59) \times \frac{\text{number of days eating fruit and vegetables in a year}}{365} \qquad (9)$$

The model estimates an individual's probability of developing hypertension. The prevalence of hypertension at the population level is then estimated by aggregating individuals' probabilities.

4 Running the Model: Validating and Intervening

4.1 Assessing Model Quality: Validation and Alternative Views

Ahrweiler and Gilbert have summarized three different views on the meaning of a simulation's quality in policy modeling [44]. The first or 'standard' view is to perform verification (ensure that the software implementation matches the model specification) and validation (ensure that the simulation's outputs *resemble* the target). Note that a perfect match between the simulation's output and the target dataset is neither required nor expected: for example, a model being a simplification of the world, it did not include all of the processes that may have shaped the observed data. The second view rejects the possibility of evaluation by considering that there is no perfect ground-truth data. That is, a dataset is a recorded *observation*, in the same way as the model's output can be deemed to be an observation. The third view notes that models can be useful without empirical support, and that their validity should be judged by its intended users. An example is Schelling's model of segregation, which became famous in the field of modeling and simulation without validation.

In this chapter, we assess the model quality using validation. This typically proceeds as follows: calibrate the model on data for year X, let the model run up to year Y under the dynamics that prevailed in that time interval for its real-world counterpart, and compare the model outcome at Y with the real-world data for this year. This highlights an important principle similar to data mining: a model is built from a dataset ('training set') that must be different from the dataset used for validation ('testing set'). In our case, we used the CHIS 2007 to calibrate the model. We will use the prevalence of hypertension in the CHIS 2012 data for validation. The model thus starts in 2007 and runs for 5 years. A 5 year incidence also makes sense in our context since hypertension is a chronic disease condition that occurs due to cumulative risk exposure. For example, the model cannot just run for a year and then be validated. As aforementioned, the simulated years should incorporate the same dynamics as really happened in Los Angeles County between 2007 and 2012 regarding hypertension. Since no large scale intervention on hypertension or healthy eating took place, we set the exogenous (intervention) γ to 0, in which case Eqs. 5 and 6 simplify to Eqs. 3 and 4. Note that γ is only set to 0 for validation (i.e. the absence of an intervention): the next section tests our virtual intervention by assigning a non-zero value to γ, in which case Eqs. 5 and 6 are used.

There are two sources of randomness when running the simulation: the initial hypertension status of each individual, which is randomly assigned based on the

Table 3 Validation starting with the observed 2007 data, simulating, and comparing to the 2012 observed data

Age	2007 observed prevalence	2012 observed prevalence		2012 simulated prevalence	
	Mean (%)	Mean (%)	95% CI	Mean (%)	95% CI
18–34	7.00	8.10	(5.40; 10.80)	8.61	(8.47; 8.75)
35–64	20.90	22.50	(19.50; 25.50)	23.88	(23.74; 24.02)
65+	52.90	54.20	(50.80; 57.50)	55.86	(55.01; 56.65)
Overall	27.09	28.45	(25.41; 31.46)	29.67	(29.30; 30.31)

baseline CHIS data; and the possibility of developing hypertension during the simulation, which is also probabilistically-driven based on CHIS data. The randomness means that, for a given node of the social network (i.e. person in the population), the event of developing hypertension might occur in one simulation run yet might not necessarily occur in a different simulation run. The simulation must thus be run multiple times to yield a mean prevalence estimate so that we do not use one possible outlier simulation run as the simulation result. The results of the validation in Table 3 are obtained by running 100 simulations and reporting the mean as well as the 95% confidence interval (CI). Results show that our mean simulated prevalence closely aligns with the observed data.

4.2 Virtual Intervention

The simulated intervention is a media campaign to promote the descriptive social norm of healthy eating, which is delivered by increasing the influence of healthier eating individuals within their existing social networks. A hypothetical well-funded and mass-reach campaign promoting the social norm that "many people are eating fruits and vegetables in your community" is applied in the adult population of LAC. The social norm to be enhanced here is the descriptive social norm instead of an injunctive norm message, since descriptive social norm has been shown to have a stronger impact on health behavior than injunctive norm message and health information messages [45]. A number of social media channels including Facebook, Twitter, Google+, Yelp, Instagram, or YouTube, are assumed to be utilized to help those with sufficient fruit and/or vegetable intake share their own healthy eating behavior within the social network, as in the case of the LAC initiative seeking to reduce sugary drink consumption [46]. We assume that only the promotion campaign takes place over the media channels. If either complementary or adversarial campaigns were simultaneously occurring, they would need to be modeled as interacting spreading phenomena [47]. The purpose is to increase the visibility of healthy eating behavior through the social networks, and ultimately increase fruit and vegetable consumption via norm change and reduce the burden of hypertension. Based

Table 4 Results of our virtual intervention

	2012 prevalence, 5% norm		2012 prevalence, 10% norm		2012 prevalence, 15% norm	
Age	Mean (%)	95% CI	Mean (%)	95% CI	Mean (%)	95% CI
18–34	8.55	(8.48; 8.57)	8.53	(8.47; 8.58)	8.49	(8.45; 8.54)
35–64	23.83	(23.77; 23.87)	23.74	(23.70; 23.79)	23.78	(23.73; 23.83)
65+	55.18	(54.93; 55.43)	55.22	(54.98; 55.47)	54.85	(54.61; 55.08)
Overall	27.09	(29.29; 29.51)	29.39	(29.28; 29.59)	29.27	(29.16; 29.38)

on studies of social norm [45] and our previous calibrations [11], we assume that the intervention enhances the healthy norm of fruit and/or vegetable consumption by 10% (i.e. $\gamma = 0.1$), which is a conservative assumption compared to the magnitude of social norm change on health behavior [28, 45, 48]. Sensitivity analyses are conducted by varying γ from 0.05 to 0.15 in order to test the robustness of our results. As in the validation, results in Table 4 are reported over 100 runs of the simulation.

The results show that implementing the intervention at a conservative estimate ($\gamma = 0.1$) will change the overall 5 year hypertension incidence by -10.85%. Specifically, the percentage change in 5 year hypertension incidence is -4.97% among people age 18–34 years old, -4.70% in people age 35–64 years old, and -21.62% among the people age 65 and above. If we take an even more conservative estimate ($\gamma = 0.05$), we observe a change of -10.08% in 5 year hypertension incidence. A less conservative estimate ($\gamma = 0.15$) leads to a percentage change of -15.50%.

5 Discussion and Conclusion

By quantifying the extent to which a health promotion intervention could benefit a defined population, simulation models built for forecasting purposes can provide insights about the long-term effectiveness of specific interventions, helping with the decision making process from a perspective of resource allocation. Our simulations show a substantial reduction in 5 year hypertension incidence with the media campaign for healthy eating, a result that remains robust across different levels of assumed effect size in norm change. At the scale of the adult population in Los Angeles County [37], this translates to averting 14,925 (assuming a 5% norm change) to 22,962 (assuming a 15% norm change) cases of hypertension for the 5 years following the hypothetical media campaign. Given the recent estimation of an annual treatment cost of hypertension ($733 per person) [49], this intervention would have saved an annual health care cost of $10,940,269 (for a 5% norm change) to $16,831,184 (for a 15% norm change) in the county of Los Angeles in 2010 dollar.

Moreover, the $733 per capita annual cost is only for the treatment of the hypertension condition, which did not take into account the cost of the diseases associated with high blood pressure including stroke, coronary heart disease, kidney diseases, etc. [22]. As a Canadian study estimated the total attributable cost of hypertension to be $2,341 per capita per year (not counting the indirect economic cost such as productivity loss) [50], we can infer that total cost savings from these averted hypertension cases will be considerably larger than the cost savings we calculated from hypertension treatment.

While it could be difficult to estimate the program cost for a media campaign aiming to change the eating norms of fruit and vegetable consumption in LAC, the reported cost of $920,000 for the 2011–2012 media campaign in LAC to reduce sugary drink consumption could give us an idea of how much the cost would be for such a campaign, which used social media and paid outdoor media on transit and billboards [46]. This budget of $920,000 for one countywide campaign, if applicable for our hypothetical media campaign to increase fruit and vegetable consumption, is between 5.5% (assuming a 15% norm change) and 8.4% (assuming a 5% norm change) of the annual saving of hypertension treatment cost, which means that this kind of norm-changing campaign can be cost-saving within 5 years.

One major limit of our paper is that the model has not yet included a module that simulates the mortality outcome for the population, and thus we have not yet explored the reduction of premature deaths due to increasing fruit and vegetable consumption. The advantage of simulating mortality outcome in relation to promoting healthier eating behavior is that it captures both the benefit of preventing hypertension (primary prevention) and the benefit of helping hypertensive people control blood pressure (secondary or tertiary prevention) [51]. We plan to include mortality outcome as well as diseases such as stroke and coronary heart diseases in our next phase of model development.

Another major limit of our paper is that we have not yet modeled the race/ethnic difference in risk of hypertension. As African Americans and non-Latino White people have different age trajectories for developing hypertension [52], it is possible that a stronger emphasis on the media campaign targeting the African American communities might reduce more hypertension burden for every dollar spent on changing eating norms. We look forward to expanding our model to incorporate the race dimension for a better understanding of the differences in health benefits associated with different targeting strategies.

It will be informative if our model outputs the annual hypertension prevalence over all the simulated calendar years, instead of simply yielding a prevalence estimate at the end of the 5 year simulated period. However, at this point our model has not developed a functional module to document the time evolution of the prevalence of hypertension. We look forward to developing the module that tracks and outputs the annual prevalence so that planners of health interventions have a clear vision of when to anticipate substantial health benefit after the implementation of the planned intervention.

The broader significance of our agent-based model lies in the fact that preventing hypertension is not the only health benefit that can result from more fruit and vegetable consumption, and fruit and vegetable consumption is not the only health behavior that can be changed by modifying social norm. Other chronic diseases that can be prevented and controlled by lifestyle modification may use norm-changing interventions, which can be assessed with a validated ABM specifically reflecting the demographic makeup of the local communities [27]. Our modeling approach, then, can be applied in topics where changing descriptive social norm is feasible in improving health outcomes and saving long-term medical expenditures.

Acknowledgements PJG wishes to thank the College of Liberal Arts & Sciences and the Department of Computer Science at Northern Illinois University for financial support.

References

1. Epstein JM (2008) J Artif Soc Soc Simul 11(4):12
2. Leischow S, Milstein B (2006) Am J Public Health 96(3):403
3. Luke DA, Stamatakis KA (2012) Annu Rev Public Health 33:357
4. Gilbert N, Troitzsch K (2005) Simulation for the social scientist. McGraw-Hill International
5. Epstein JM (2009) Nature 460:687
6. Giabbanelli PJ (2013) A novel framework for complex networks and chronic diseases. Springer, Berlin, Heidelberg, pp 207–215
7. Nianogo R, Onyebuchi A (2015) Am J Public Health 105(3):e20
8. Cavana RY, Clifford LV (2006) Syst Dyn Rev 22(4):321
9. Levy D, Mabry P, Wang Y, Gortmaker S, Huang T, Marsh T, Moodie M, Swinburn B (2010) Obes Rev 12:378
10. Verigin T, Giabbanelli PJ, Davidsen PI (2016) In: Proceedings of the 49th annual simulation symposium 2016 (ANSS'16), pp 9:1–9:10
11. Giabbanelli PJ, Alimadad A, Dabbaghian V, Finegood DT (2012) J Comput Sci 3(1):17
12. Zhang D, Giabbanelli PJ, Arah O, Zimmerman F (2014) Am J Public Health 104(7):1217
13. Giabbanelli PJ, Crutzen R (2017) Comput Math Methods Med 2017:5742629
14. Deck P, Giabbanelli P, Finegood D (2013) Can J Diabetes 37:S269
15. Auchincloss AH, Riolo RL, Brown DG, Cook J, Roux AVD (2011) Am J Prev Med 40(3):303
16. Lieberman M, Gauvin L, Bukowski W, White D (2001) Eat Behav 2(3):215
17. Klesges R, Bartsch D, Norwood J, Kautzrnan D, Haugrud S (1984) Int J Eat Disord 3(4):35
18. Rivis A, Sheeran P (2002) Curr Psychol 22(2):218
19. Stok F, Ridder D, Vet E, Wit J (2014) Br J Health Psychol 19(1):52
20. Wakefield M, Loken B, Hornik R (2010) Lancet 376(9748):1261
21. Wang L, Manson J, Gaziano J, Buring J, Sesso H (2012) Am J Hypertens 25(2):180
22. Mozaffarian D, Benamin E, Go A et al (2015) Circulation p. CIR. 0000000000000350
23. Sacks F, Svetkey L, Vollmer W et al (2001) N Engl J Med 344(1):3
24. CDC (2016) Badges and widgets. http://www.cdc.gov/nccdphp/dch/multimedia/badges.htm
25. Porter K, Curtin L, Carroll M, Li X, Smon M, Fielding J (2011) Natl Health Stat Rep 42
26. Dixon H, Scully M, Wakefield M, White V, Crawford D (2007) Soc Sci Med 65(7):1311
27. Li Y, Lawley M, Siscovick D, Zhang D, Pagan J (2016) Prev Chronic Dis 13:E59
28. Li Y, Zhang D, Pagan J (2016) J Urban Health 1–12
29. Giabbanelli PJ, Jackson PJ, Finegood DT (2014) Modelling the joint effect of social determinants and peers on obesity among Canadian adults, pp 145–160

30. Grimm V, Berger U, DeAngelis DL, Polhill JG, Giske J, Railsback SF (2010) Ecol Model 221(23):2760
31. National Cancer Institute Health Behaviors Research Branch (2007) Food attitudes and behavior (FAB) survey
32. Hsiao C (1996) Logit and probit models, pp 410–428
33. Comellas F, Ozn J, Peters JG (2000) Inf Process Lett 76(1):83
34. Giabbanelli PJ (2011) Adv Complex Syst 14(06):853
35. Giabbanelli PJ (2010) In: 2010 IEEE globecom workshops, pp 389–393
36. Zimmerman F (2013) Soc Sci Med 3(80):47
37. Ponce N, Lavarreda S, Yen W, Brown E, DiSogra C, Satter D (2014) Public Health Rep 119(4):388
38. Barriere L, Comellas F, Dalfo C, Fiol M (2016) J Phys A: Math Theor 49(22):225202
39. Casagrande SS, Wang Y, Anderson C, Gary T (2007) Am J Prev Med 32(4):257
40. Gregorio JD, Lee J (2002) Rev Income Wealth 48(3):395
41. Powell L, Auld M, Chaloupka F, O'Malley P, Johnston L (2007) Adv Health Econ Health Serv Res 17:23
42. Beydoun M, Powell L, Wang Y (2008) Soc Sci Med 66(11):2218
43. Rodriguez B, Labarthe D, Huang B, Lopez-Gomez J (1994) Hypertension 24(6):779
44. Ahrweiler P, Gilbert N (2015) The quality of social simulation: an example from research policy modelling, pp 35–55
45. Robinson E, Fleming A, Higgs S (2014) Health Psychol 33(9):1057
46. Barragan N, Noller A, Robles B, Gase L, Leighs M, Bogert S, Simon P, Kuo T (2013) Health Promot Pract 15(2):208
47. Patel I, Nguyen H, Belyi E, Getahun Y, Abdulkareem S, Giabbanelli PJ, Mago V (2017) In: SoutheastCon 2017, pp 1–8
48. Zhang X, Cowling D, Tang H (2010) Tob Control 19(S1):i51
49. Davis K (2013) Expenditures for hypertension among adults age 18 and older, 2010: estimates for the US civilian noninstitutionalized population
50. Weaver C, Clement F, Campbell N, James M et al (2015) Hypertension 66(3):502
51. Conlin P, Chow D, Miller E, Svetkey L, Lin P, Harsha D, Moore T, Sacks F, Appel L (2000) Am J Hypertens
52. Hertz R, Unger A, Cornell J, Saunders E (2005) Arch Intern Med 165(18):2098

Soft Data Analytics with Fuzzy Cognitive Maps: Modeling Health Technology Adoption by Elderly Women

Noshad Rahimi, Antonie J. Jetter, Charles M. Weber and Katherine Wild

Abstract Modeling how patients adopt personal health technology is a challenging problem: Decision-making processes are largely unknown, occur in complex, multi-stakeholder settings, and may play out differently for different products and users. To address this problem, this chapter develops a soft analytics approach, based on Fuzzy Cognitive Maps (FCM) that leads to adoption models that are specific for a particular product and group of adopters. Its empirical grounding is provided by a case study, in which a group of women decides whether to adopt a wearable remote healthcare monitoring device. The adoption model can simulate different product configurations and levels of support and provide insight as to what scenarios will most likely lead to successful adoption. The model can be used by product developers and rollout managers to support technology planning decisions.

1 Introduction

Health technology adoption is a challenging problem for product developers because many of the intended users of health technology devices tend not to adopt. Glucose self-monitoring technology, for example, is relatively inexpensive, widely available, and easy-to-use, but many patients fail to monitor their blood sugar

N. Rahimi (✉) · A. J. Jetter · C. M. Weber
Department of Engineering and Technology Management, Portland State University,
Portland, OR, USA
e-mail: noshad@pdx.edu

A. J. Jetter
e-mail: jettera@pdx.edu

C. M. Weber
e-mail: webercm@pdx.edu

K. Wild
Oregon Center for Aging & Technology, Oregon Health & Science University,
Portland, OR, USA
e-mail: wildk@ohsu.edu

© Springer International Publishing AG, part of Springer Nature 2018
P. J. Giabbanelli et al. (eds.), *Advanced Data Analytics in Health*, Smart Innovation,
Systems and Technologies 93, https://doi.org/10.1007/978-3-319-77911-9_4

frequently enough to prevent long-term disease effects [1]. Similarly, up to 50% of patients suffering from obstructive sleep apnea reject the use of recommended CACP (continuous positive airway pressure) devices or stop using them within a week [2], even though untreated sleep apnea decreases life expectancy. Remote Health Monitoring Technologies (RHMT) for the elderly can facilitate independent living in the family home, which 90% of them prefer over living in care facilities [3]. Yet, the elderly are slow to adopt these technologies [4] for reasons that may be related to the natural consequences of aging, the complexity of the healthcare context [5] and the adoption process itself [6]. Product developers consequently want to know what motivates a consumer to adopt a health technology, what features are desired, and which roll-out strategies are likely to improve and sustain technology use.

To address these questions from a practical perspective, we present a mixed-method approach for modeling health technology adoption with FCM that combines qualitative data acquisition with quantitative analytical models. The method is demonstrated with a case study on the adoption of RHMT by elderly women because they are frequently reluctant to adopt new technology [7]. Our method returns to the foundation of FCMs in dealing with the vagueness inherent to quality data, collected through ethnographic interviews and examined via text analysis. This makes it possible to develop product and adopter-specific recommendations for fostering health technology adoption, which is useful for health product and health technology planning.

The chapter is structured as follows. Section 2.1 discusses the challenge of technology adoption among the elderly and outlines the need for new modeling and decision-making approaches. Section 2.2 introduces FCM and Sect. 2.3 provides a brief state of the art of FCM in the context of technology adoption planning. Section 3 provides an overview over the approach taken in this work and introduces the case study. Section 4 presents results. Section 5 discusses findings and avenues for future research.

2 Technical Background

2.1 Health Technology Adoption by the Elderly

Remote health monitoring technologies (RHMT), such as wearable activity trackers and in-home monitoring systems, can contribute to a solution by allowing elderly to live independently. They can improve the management of chronic conditions and thus reduce the occurrence of crisis situations; improve the assessment of care needs in emergency and everyday situations; and free up caregiver schedules by enabling remote check-ins, visits, and data exchange with healthcare providers [8]. Moreover, the sensors embedded in RHMT efficiently create hard data (rather than self-reports) on behaviors and physiological responses. These can be tracked over weeks, months, or years and combined with other datasets, such as data on med-ications. This is expected to help advance medical research [9]. Accordingly, the potential benefits of RHMT motivate a large body of national (e.g. [10]) and international (e.g. [11]) research.

Theories on health technology adoption are fragmented, and their ability to model actual adoption behavior is very limited [12]. A case in point is the Unified Theory of Acceptance and Use of Technology (UTAUT), which the literature sees as a solid foundation for the study of elderly health technology adoption [13]. The theory tries to explain how four key input constructs—usefulness, ease of use, social influence and facilitating conditions—affect the intention to adopt and the actual adoption rate. However, the concepts in the UTAUT are too general to provide actionable insights for specific health contexts for three reasons. (*1*) *Lack of Specificity*: The factors mean different things to different technology users [14] and need to be understood within the specific use context. (*2*) *Lack of Stakeholder Involvement*: Healthcare is a complex, multi-stakeholder setting in which tech-nology users are influenced by medical professionals, informal caregivers who serve as technology gatekeepers, and insurance providers. UTAUT does not con-sider these complexities [6]. (*3*) *Data scarcity*: applying UTAUT for planning processes requires data. However, data on key factors of the elderly decision-making process is scarce: the process is largely internal and is researched with qualitative techniques. Existing data is thus subject to interpretation and specific to a particular time and context, and it may not apply to a different product, user, or time.

This work uses a mixed-method approach for modeling health technology adoption. It builds on UTAUT, using the factors identified by the theory, and investigates their meaning and importance in the context of a specific health technology. The approach's backbone is FCM, which serves as a data acquisition and modeling method.

2.2 Fuzzy Cognitive Maps

Fuzzy Cognitive Maps [15] are signed directed graphs: they consist of nodes, so-called "concepts" that are connected through arrows that show the direction of influence between concepts. A positive (negative) arrow pointing from concept A to concept B indicates that concept A causally increases (decreases) concept B. Weights can be assigned to reflect the strength of the connections. Concepts are typically verbally described and can contain hard-to-quantify concepts, such as "usefulness".

Structurally, FCMs are digraphs. As such, graph theoretical concepts apply and metrics such as density (an index of connectivity), "degree centrality (number of links incident to a given concept node)" and indegree and outdegree (the direction of the arrows) are frequently used [16] to describe the overall structure of the model, as well as the position of specific concepts in the network. A high out-degree (a relatively larger number of outbound arrows than other concepts), for example, is assumed to hint at the importance of the concept as an influencer/leverage in the system.

Computationally, FCMs are regarded as a simple form of recursive neural networks [17]. Concepts are equivalent to neurons, but other than neurons, they are not either "on" (= 1) or "off" (= 0 or −1), but can take states in-between and are therefore "fuzzy". Fuzzy concepts are non-linear functions that transform the path-weighted activations directed towards them (their "causes") into a value in [0, 1] or [−1, 1]. When a neuron "fires" (i.e., when a concept changes its state), it affects all concepts that are causally dependent upon it. Depending on the direction and size of this effect, and on the threshold levels of the dependent concepts, the affected concepts may subsequently change their state as well, thus activating further concepts within the network. Because FCMs allow feedback loops, newly activated concepts can influence concepts that have already been activated before. As a result, the activation spreads in a non-linear fashion through the FCM net until the system reaches a stable limit cycle or fixed point. FCM calculation models the spreading activation through the network by multiplying a vector of causal activation C_{t-1} with the square connection matrix E derived from the FCM graph. $S(x)$ is a squashing function:

$$C_t = S(C_{t-1} \times E) \tag{1}$$

Commonly used squashing functions, such as bivalent, trivalent or logistic function restrict the concept states to discrete final states, such as $\{0, 1\}$ or $\{-1, 0, 1\}$ or to intervals $[-1; 1]$ or $[0; 1]$. Bivalent squashing functions can represent an increase of a concept, trivalent functions can represent an increase or a decrease of a concept and logistic functions can represent the degree of an increase of decrease of a concept [18]. A commonly used logistic function is a hyperbolic tangent function:

$$S(c_{it}) = \tanh(\lambda c_{it}) = \frac{e^{\lambda c_{it}} - e^{-\lambda c_{it}}}{e^{\lambda c_{it}} + e^{-\lambda c_{it}}} \tag{2}$$

λ is a constant that defines the slope. For $\lambda = 1$ the squashing function is almost linear, which means that gradual concepts changes only have gradual impacts on other concepts. Also, inputs in the interval $[-1; 1]$ do not map to outputs in the same range but only to approximately 80% of the maximum and minimum values, so that final concepts states are never at the extremes. For $\lambda = 5$, hyperbolic tangent approximates a full normalization into the interval $[-1; 1]$ [19].

Concepts that are persistent over multiple iterations (e.g. knowledge remains available after it was first acquired), rather than one-time shocks to the system (e.g. a terrorist attack), are 'clamped', which means they are reset to their initial value after each iteration.

All FCMs have "meta-rules": several input vectors—so-called input regions—lead to the same final system state [20]. FCMs with continuous concept states, so-called "continuous-state machines" can result in chaotic behavior [20]. FCMs with discrete concept states, so-called "finite state machines" result in either a fixed state vector or in a limit cycle between a number of fixed state vectors [20, 21]. At this point, any new iteration delivers the same result as the prior iteration or the difference between the iterations is considered negligible because it falls under a predefined threshold for stability, epsilon (ε). The number of iterations it takes until a stable fixed point or limited cycle is reached depends on squashing functions, initial state, and the structure of the FCM [16, 18, 19, 22]. The stable end states of concepts cannot be interpreted in absolute terms, but only relative to other factors in the system or relative to other system descriptions.

2.3 FCM Modeling and Simulation

FCMs [15] evolved from cognitive maps, which were developed by social scientists to capture and analyze decision-makers cognition. Cognitive maps are mental models that represent the subjective causal knowledge of decision-makers, which is acquired through social, experiential, and formal learning and is therefore unique to each decision-maker, though members of the same group often share similar cognitive maps [16]. Cognitive maps can contain misconceptions, oversimplifications, and mistakes, which can result in poor decision-making. Their value to researchers is their ability to help explain how a decision-maker thinks and what he/she will likely do, even if these actions run counter to facts or logic [17]. FCMs enhance this analysis by allowing researchers to draw dynamic inferences from a cognitive map and computationally answer "what if" questions through simulation. Accordingly, FCMs were first used to research decision-makers' worldviews, as well as to support decisions when "hard" data is not available and models have to be based on expert judgment [18]. These type of applications still exist in Future Studies, where FCM are used to create scenarios [19], and in Environmental Modelling, where FCM elicit the reasoning of individuals who have a "stake in the problem" and their likely response to policy alternatives [23]. A lot of FCM research, however, applies "hard" analytical approaches and constructs FCM models from data [20]. We take a different path and emphasize the qualitative roots of FCM by analyzing subjective, verbal data, and by employing methods for qualitative analysis to create FCM simulation models.

In technology adoption, this type of work has been done in educational [24], agricultural [25], and healthcare organizational settings [25]. However, none of these studies address health technology adoption in the personal realm (vs. healthcare or other organizations). Moreover, the studies do not *model adoption outcomes as an FCM*. Instead, they use FCM as a data acquisition tool to identify barriers and benefits of the technology that may influence adoption without simulating the actual adoption [21], or to create inputs for the Bass adoption model [22]. Going beyond this state-of-the-art, we model how the generally recognized factors for technology adoption (according to UTAUT) impact adoption by a specific set of stakeholders in a specific adoption setting. The resulting FCM model can be used to simulate which combination of factors leads to higher or lower adoption outcomes. These insights help technology planners modify product features and roll-out strategies in ways that increase adoption. We thus address the three challenges identified above, namely the need for data, the need for specificity, and the need for stakeholder involvement.

3   Method

While our method is intended for any multi-stakeholder health technology adoption process to which UTAUT applies, we develop and test it in a specific context: the adoption of a wearable fall detector, named Product X, by a group of elderly women. Study participants were the elderly adopters and their technology gate-keepers, such as children or informal caregivers, who influence the adoption decision [26]. We, therefore, discuss the case study setting and the method concurrently.

3.1   Case Study Setting

The study was conducted in collaboration with ORCATECH—the Oregon Center for Aging and Technology (NIA grant, P30AG024978). ORCATECH researches the clinical implications of technologies for the aging population and regularly conducts field tests of RHMT products, such as Product X, a prototype wristwatch with fall detection capability (NIH contract R44AG032160-03). ORCATECH selected the participants for the field test from its 'Living Laboratory' panel of elderly volunteers. We selected the four participants for our FCM study from the field test cohort based on gender (only elderly women and female caregivers) and practical concerns, namely the willingness of the elderly women and their caregivers to participate in a parallel study.[1]

3.2   Method Overview

Data Collection: Cognitive maps were collected from two elderly women and their two caregivers in separate face-to-face interviews, which implemented the principles of ethnographic techniques [27]. These principles include (1) making the

---

[1]Detail research material can be found on OSF website (Springer Chapter book: Rahimi et al.): https://osf.io/hp7r2/

interview purpose explicit and known to participants, (2) repeatedly offering explanations to the participants, (3) recording participant explanations and asking follow-up questions, (4) acknowledging researcher's lack of knowledge about participants' personal perspectives, and (5) using participants' everyday language. The interviews took place in the participants' homes at the beginning of the field test of Product X, when the prototypes were first deployed. The elderly women were asked to subjectively define and expand on the constructs of UTAUT, based on their own perception. The caregivers were asked to provide their knowledge about the UTAUT concepts and connections that matter to the person for whom they care. Responses were audio recorded and documented as a cognitive map, using Mental Modeler software. Participants were encouraged to review and improve upon the map during the interview, which was concluded when the participant that there was nothing else to add.

Analysis of Interview Data: Four separate maps resulted from the four interviews. Each map was refined to reflect additional data from the audio recordings and subsequently merged with the maps from the other participants. Similar to [16], this process built on qualitative analysis techniques: All recordings were coded in Atlas.ti (a software tool for qualitative analysis from atlasti.com). During open coding, concepts, and their higher level categories emerged (formed as code families), using predominantly the language of the participant. During the subsequent second coding step (axial coding), these concepts and their causal relations were generalized into broader code families. During the final step, selective coding, the remaining codes were further refined to represent generalizable constructs and then standardized across all maps [28]. During each step, cognitive maps were updated. In total, seven maps with standardized concept labels and meanings were generated: one map each for the two elderly women (W1 and W2) and their gatekeepers (G1 and G2), based on interview data; one map each for both elderly/caregiver pairs (W1/G1 and W2/G2), based on a combination of their individual maps, and, finally, an integrated map that combines insights gained from both elderly/caregiver maps (W1/G1/W2/G2). To preserve the insights from all participants, integration was done additively: if a concept or connection occurred in any one of the contributing maps it was included, even if other contributing maps had omitted it. This integration is a complex process [29], which has become possible through the power of qualitative aggregation [16]. Here, using Atlas.ti, all the open-codes that grouped and formed code families (i.e. the standardized concepts) are organized and preserved. The accumulated codes from all the interviews provide the information base from which the best abstract concepts and corresponding links are extracted. Weights for causal connections were assigned in 0.25 increments from -1 to $= 1$. This was done separately for each pair of maps (W1/G1 and W2/G2), based on the emphasis of both participants. Thus, the edge weights were assigned based on evidence from the semantics and the frequencies of the related qualitative codes that had emerged from the interviews. For example, using Atlas.ti data on the coded audio, 1 was assigned when both participants strongly emphasized the connection and 0.25 were assigned when both participants provided low emphasis, or one participant provided medium emphasis but the other participant did not report on the connection at all. The process was repeated for the integration map (W1/G1/W2/G2). The resulting weighted cognitive map represents the collective knowledge of all participants.

Like other studies (e.g. [16]), this research has not used a fuzzy set for weight assignment. However, future research could benefit from using a fuzzy set.

FCM Modeling and Analysis: the weighted cognitive map was implemented as an FCM model. To test it, the model was run with participant-specific input vectors that reflect their judgments regarding product characteristics and contextual factors (e.g. social support, facilitating conditions), which were obtained in post-adoption interviews after the completion of the Product X field test. Given these inputs, the model foresaw that neither participant would adopt the product after the trial, even if it was given to her free of charge. This was correct. The tested model was analyzed to obtain data on (1) on the structure of the participant-provided model of technology adoption, such as density, centrality of concepts, and system drivers and (2) data on the dynamic behavior of the FCM model in response to various input scenarios. The findings of this analysis are reported in the subsequent case study section.

4 Case Study Results: Modeling Technology Adoption with FCM

4.1 Structure and Content of the Model

The integrated FCM model (W1/G1/W2/G2) consists of 52 unique concepts with 105 connections. It has a density (links/concepts) of 0.04, which is similar to other studies in which stakeholders model complex issues with many concepts [30]. It is, however, low in comparison to expert-designed FCM models, which typically contain significantly fewer concepts [31]. The model is thus likely holistic, rather than reductionist.

Figure 1 illustrates the overall structure of the model. As can be seen by the cluster of arrows, the three concepts with the highest indegree (the number of arrows pointing to the concept) and degree (the number of arrows connected to the concept) are Perceived Usefulness (15 and 18), Social Influence (9, 15), and Perceived Ease of Use (8, 10), which are the main constructs of the UTAUT. The right-hand side of the model also reflects the key structure of UTAUT: Perceived Usefulness, Perceived Ease of Use and Social Influence impact the intention to adopt, which causes people to adopt if favorable facilitating conditions are in place. These factors are "unpacked" into a large number of causal factors. For the most part, the model thus confirms (but provides contextual detail) to UTAUT. However, there are important differences: Because of the statistical methods in use, most research on UTAUT assumes that the factors contributing to usefulness, ease of use

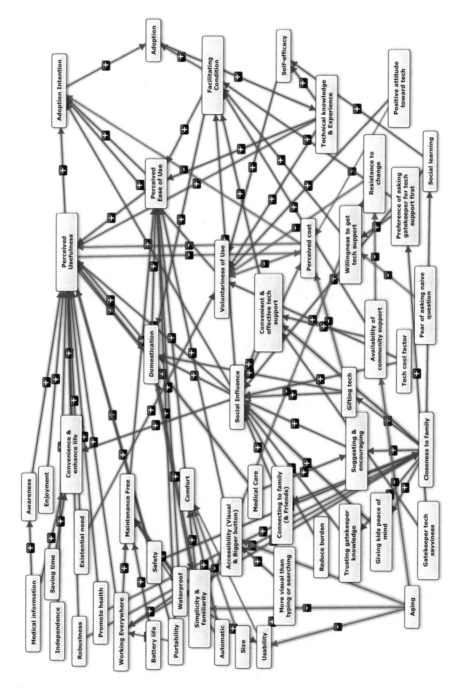

Fig. 1 Overall model structure (the model is accessible on: https://osf.io/hp7r2/)

and social influence are distinct, yet the model shows that the same factor (e.g. portability of the device) can contribute to several of these concepts (i.e. usefulness and ease of use) and thus impact overall adoption through more than one pathway. The participant's model shows interdependencies between core UTAUT constructs (e.g. ease of use causes usefulness to increase) and feedback cycles (e.g. domestication → ease of use → usefulness → domestication). By modeling these phenomena holistically, the FCM can reflect far-reaching and indirect effects.

Perceived Usefulness has the highest degree centrality of all concepts in the model (18). It impacts adoption by increasing adoption intention, reducing the perceived cost of the technology, and supporting the process of technology domestication (i.e. frequent engagement with technology until it becomes a part of everyday life), and creating convenience and improved quality of life as a result of technology use. Social influence occurs through many pathways, which include gatekeepers who serve as role models for technology use, give technology as a gift and thus reduce costs, and ask the elderly to use RHMT for the family's peace of mind. Gatekeepers provide low-barrier technology support, which is important because the elderly are reluctant to ask strangers for help (e.g. on a hotline).

To validate the resulting FCM model (in Fig. 1), we simulated the model based on the base data set gathered from the participants during the pre-adoption data collection. The base data contained the elderly women's perceptions of the device they tried in relation to the main constructs of UTAUT (usefulness, ease of use, social influence and facilitating conditions). Then, we compared the suggested outcomes of the model with the actual outcomes that we gathered in the post-adoption data collection. In both cases, our FCM model was able to successfully predict the adoption outcome. The simulation results were in line with the actual adoption behavior (obtained in the post-adoption data collection); hence the model is validated.

4.2   Simulation: Model Interpretations and Implications

The model shows that technology adoption is impacted by those factors on which product developers traditionally focus namely product characteristics and facilitating conditions. In addition, they are affected by factors that are largely beyond the control of product companies, namely social support by family members and other gatekeepers. Can a good technology product make up for unfavorable social support, i.e. can we expect technology adoption by a growing number of isolated elderly [32]? And can gatekeeper support make up for the quirks and drawbacks of emergent RHMT, which is not yet fully mature [23]?

We explored these questions by simulating adoption outcomes in response to different combinations of feature sets and social support. We ran seven scenarios, which are reported in Table 1. In the first four scenarios, we assumed an average ("good enough") product that was usable but had some flaws, and we vary the influence of the social support. The product was based on participant feedback and

Table 1 Simulation results (All simulations run with hyperbolic tangent [37] and clamping of concepts [15]; [a]*gk* stands for gatekeeper; [b]all concepts of the model are stable with an epsilon of 0.0001); The initial value for every other concepts is zero

Scenario number and description	1. OK product but no support	2. OK product with strong gk[a] support	3. OK product but lower gk[a] support (0.25)	4. OK product but little gk[a] support (0.1)	5. Better product but little gk[a] support	6. Better product with no gk[a] support	7. Better product with community training
Input concepts							
Working everywhere	0.7	0.7	0.7	0.7	0.8	0.8	0.8
Robustness	0.7	0.7	0.7	0.7	0.8	0.8	0.8
Promote health	0.7	0.7	0.7	0.7	0.8	0.8	0.8
Closeness to family	0	1	0.25	0.1	0.1	0	0
Gatekeeper tech savviness	0	1	0.25	0.1	0.1	0	0
Fear of asking naïve question	1	0	0.75	0.9	0.9	1	0
Availability of community support	0	0	0	0	0	0	1
Output concepts							
Usefulness	0.46	0.79	0.69	0.59	0.63	0.51	0.55
Ease of use	0.08	0.59	0.45	0.28	0.29	0.09	0.18
Adoption intention	0.32	0.86	0.73	0.56	0.58	0.35	0.44
Adoption	**0.16**	**0.67**	**0.51**	**0.35**	**0.36**	**0.17**	**0.28**
Stability iteration[b]	15	9	12	14	17	18	16

suggested improvements after the Product X trial. It was configured as follows: medium operating range (i.e. works in the house but not at the far end of the yard), works reliably, and has features that promote healthy behaviors (e.g. step counter). The activation values for the concepts "works everywhere", "robustness", and "promotes health" are 0.7 in each scenario. In the baseline scenario 1 (no social support and hence high fear of asking a naïve question), this resulted in a useful but not comfortable product and a really low adoption intention and adoption. Scenario 2 reflects strong positive social influence by gatekeepers, who can provide encouragement, and facilitate the use of technology. These gatekeepers were family members who had technology knowledge of their own (gatekeeper tech savviness +1).

The elderly felt close to them and interacted with them frequently during visits and phone calls (closeness to family +1) and had no fear of asking naïve question. Scenario 2 resulted in the highest adoption intention and adoption. We also explored the effect of lower social support situations with lower gatekeeper support and expertise (tested with 0.25 in scenario 3 and 0.1 in scenario 4). Respectively, the lower the social support, the higher the fear of asking naïve question is, since elderly now has to rely on other people to answer her questions. Both these scenarios predict lower adoption outcomes (lower with less social support).

We subsequently tested if strong product features offset low levels of gatekeeper support: so in scenario 5, we modified scenario 4 to reflect improved product features. This resulted in a slightly higher adoption intention and adoption than scenario 4. However, adoption lagged far behind the adoption of a *less* attractive product, but with moderate levels of gatekeeper support and expertise (scenario 2).

In scenario 6, we simulated the adoption of the better product without any social support. This resulted in a very low adoption outcome, suggesting that improvements to the product do not increase the chances of adoption as effectively as social support does. So, to some extent, gatekeeper support can compensate for product features. In our post-adoption interviews, participants confirmed this finding. They reported that family support not only helps them use technology that they find difficult to understand—it is the main driver of their adoption decision.

A potential drawback of our FCM model could be a lack of flexibility, which may make it impossible to simulate the outcomes of innovative product designs or roll-out strategies that were unknown at the model building stage. To allow for this possibility, we modeled an intervention that is proposed in the literature but did not occur in the Product X trial, namely the use of community trainers, who can provide culturally sensitive, jargon-free, and low-barrier support [24]. Such trainers are expected to help overcome the adoption gap for elderly without family support who, arguably, would benefit most from RHMT. In scenario 7, we modeled the use of community trainers by setting a nonzero value to "Availability of community support". As suggested in the FCM model in Fig. 1, this concept increases "Convenient & effective tech support" and "Facilitating Condition" while decreasing "Resistance to change". Scenario 7 shows a rate of adoption that is higher than that in scenario 6, yet lower than that in the family gatekeeper scenario. This is likely a realistic outcome: even a well-designed training service likely cannot provide the multitude of functions that family or a friend's social support provides.

5   Discussion and Conclusion

This chapter demonstrates a soft analytics method, which contextualizes theoretical insights from health technology adoption by combining ethnographic interviews and FCM. It involves stakeholders, overcomes data scarcity, and provides specificity to health technology adoption theory. The empirical grounding for this method is provided by a case study, in which women decide whether to adopt a wearable remote healthcare monitoring device. Our work shows that the model can simulate adoption outcomes, given different features and levels of social support. It can help decision-makers in healthcare product and technology development identify suitable feature sets and roll-out strategies, based on a deep understanding of the dynamics of their product's specific adoption process. In addition to these practical contributions, the work contributes to addressing the current paucity of FCMs built using qualitative technique. Thus, it brings FCM research back to its origins of cognitive mapping. We also contribute to technology adoption research by translating abstract theoretical insights into models that represent a specific case. In doing so, we demonstrate the importance of technology gatekeepers in the adoption process, which current health research addresses only insufficiently.

As a demonstration project, our work is subject to limitations, which can be overcome by further research. First, we synthesize our insights from only four participants and thus from a much smaller number of respondents than is common in qualitative user or marketing research, as well as in some other FCM studies: They [16] report theme saturation after 20–30 participants, at which point additional interviews do not provide new concepts or causal connections. However, our approach is applicable to similar and even larger numbers of participants, as demonstrated by other studies, such as [33], which resulted in an integrated FCM model, based on ethnographic interviews with 69 participants. However, in even larger studies, data acquisition is certainly a bottleneck: interviews are time-consuming, as are multiple rounds of coding and re-coding, which are needed to capture the breadth of insights while also standardizing concept meanings. Several researchers are currently working on online-based data acquisition tools for FCM [29, 34]. While they will likely not replicate the exploratory depth of skilled ethnographic interviewing and analysis, these approaches may prove to be very useful in increasing the number of study participants once an initial set of concepts and connections have been identified. This will make it possible to scale FCM projects to more participants.

A second limitation of our works stems from its focus: Our model and simulation scenarios were designed to enhance our understanding of the role of the informal gatekeeper and on his/her impact on adoption, given different product feature sets. Future research may also want to include formal gatekeepers, such as healthcare professionals. These gatekeepers, according to comments during our ethnographic interviews, are to exert influence on the elderly adopter, as well as on the informal gatekeepers and peers of the elderly. To achieve a better understanding of technology adoption among a group of elderly and gatekeepers, this interplay of influence can be modeled by combining FCM and agent-based modeling, as proposed by [35]: The elderly, their informal gatekeepers and medical professionals can each be represented by group-specific FCM that encode the behavior of the agents. The agent-based model defines the rules of interactions between the agents, thus shaping an artificial market [36].

A third limitation of this study is its still limited analysis of FCM dynamics, given different inputs. Future work can explore tradeoffs between different features, the impact of different training interventions, and outcomes that are contingent upon social support provided at different stages of the adoption process. By uncovering these fundamental dynamics of technology adoption, this follow-up research could enhance the ability of analysts of big data (e.g. tracked RMHT usage data) to ascribe meaning to their analyses.

References

1. Delamater AM (2006) Improving patient adherence. Clin. Diabetes 24:71–77
2. Engleman HM, Wild MR (2003) Improving CPAP use by patients with the sleep apnoea/hypopnoea syndrome (SAHS). Sleep Med Rev 7:81–99
3. Teegardin K. Why and when to use home care for seniors. https://www.seniorliving.org/lifestyles/home-care/
4. Bowers LA. Remote patient-monitoring technology still faces reimbursement roadblock. http://www.ltlmagazine.com/article/remote-patient-monitoring-technology-still-faces-reimbursement-roadblock
5. Morgan DL (1998) Practical strategies for combining qualitative and quantitative methods: applications to health research. Qual Health Res 8:362–376
6. Crosby R, Noar SM (2010) Theory development in health promotion: are we there yet? J Behav Med 33:259–263 (2010)
7. Saborowski M, Kollak I (2014) "How do you care for technology?"–Care professionals' experiences with assistive technology in care of the elderly. Technol Forecast Soc Chang
8. Litan RE (2008) Vital signs via broadband: remote health monitoring transmits savings, enhances lives. Better Health Care Together
9. Stankovic JA, Cao Q, Doan T, Fang L, He Z, Kiran R, Lin S, Son S, Stoleru R, Wood A (2005) Wireless sensor networks for in-home healthcare: potential and challenges. In: High confidence medical device software and systems (HCMDSS) workshop
10. HealthCare Manager. Remote medication and health plan support system. https://www.sbir.gov/sbirsearch/detail/370285
11. Celler BG, Sparks R, Nepal S, Alem L, Varnfield M, Li J, Jang-Jaccard J, McBride SJ, Jayasena R (2014) Design of a multi-site multi-state clinical trial of home monitoring of chronic disease in the community in Australia. BMC Public Health 14 (2014)
12. Wagner N, Hassanein K, Head M (2010) Computer use by older adults: a multi-disciplinary review. Comput Hum Behav 26:870–882
13. Rahimi N, Jetter A (2015) Explaining health technology adoption: past, present, future. In: 2015 Portland international conference on management of engineering and technology (PICMET). IEEE, pp 2465–2495
14. Bagozzi RP (2007) The legacy of the technology acceptance model and a proposal for a paradigm shift. J Assoc Inf Syst 8:3
15. Kosko B (1986) Fuzzy cognitive maps. Int J Man-Mach Stud 24:65–75
16. Özesmi U, Özesmi SL (2004) Ecological models based on people's knowledge: a multi-step fuzzy cognitive mapping approach. Ecol Model 176:43–64
17. Dubois DJ, Prade H, Yager RR, Kosko B (2014) Adaptive inference in fuzzy knowledge networks. In: Readings in fuzzy sets for intelligent systems. Morgan Kaufmann (2014)
18. Tsadiras AK (2008) Comparing the inference capabilities of binary, trivalent and sigmoid fuzzy cognitive maps. Inf Sci 178:3880–3894
19. Bueno S, Salmeron JL (2009) Benchmarking main activation functions in fuzzy cognitive maps. Expert Syst Appl 36:5221–5229
20. Dickerson J, Kosko B (1994) Virtual worlds as fuzzy dynamical systems. In: Sheu B (ed) Technology for multimedia. IEEE Press, pp 1–35

21. Stach W, Kurgan L, Pedrycz W, Reformat M (2005) Genetic learning of fuzzy cognitive maps. Fuzzy Sets Syst 153:371–401
22. Jetter AJM (2006) Fuzzy cognitive maps in engineering and technology mangement—what works in practice? In: Anderson T, Daim T, Kocaoglu D (eds) Technology management for the global future: Proceedings of PICMET 2006, Istanbul, Turkey July, 2006
23. Jetter AJ, Sperry RC (2013) Fuzzy cognitive maps for product planning: using stakeholder knowledge to achieve corporate responsibility. In: 2013 46th Hawaii international conference on system sciences (HICSS). IEEE, pp 925–934
24. Hossain S, Brooks L (2008) Fuzzy cognitive map modelling educational software adoption. Comput Educ 51:1569–1588
25. McRoberts N, Franke AC et al (2008) A diffusion model for the adoption of agricultural innovations in structured adopting populations
26. Rahimi N, Jetter A, Weber CM (2016) An inductive ethnographic study in elderly woman technology adoption and the role of her children. In: Management of engineering and technology (PICMET). IEEE, pp 3196–3207
27. Kosko B (1988) Hidden patterns in combined and adaptive knowledge networks. Int J Approx Reason 2:377–393
28. Carley K (1993) Coding choices for textual analysis: a comparison of content analysis and map analysis. Sociol Methodol 23:75–126
29. Giabbanelli PJ, Tawfik AA (2017) Overcoming the PBL assessment challenge: design and development of the incremental thesaurus for assessing causal maps (ITACM) | SpringerLink. Springer
30. Johnson-Laird PN (1983) Mental models: towards a cognitive science of language, inference, and consciousness. In: Cognitive science series 6. Harvard University Press, Mass
31. Axelrod R (1976) Structure of decision: the cognitive maps of political elites. Princeton University Press, Princeton, NJ
32. Giabbanelli PJ, Torsney-Weir T, Mago VK (2012) A fuzzy cognitive map of the psychosocial determinants of obesity. Appl Soft Comput 12:3711–3724
33. Jenson R, Petri A, Jetter A, Gotto G, Day AR (2018) Participatory modeling with fuzzy cognitive maps: studying veterans' perspectives on access and participation in higher education. In: Innovations in collaborative modeling: transformations in higher education: The Scholarship of Engagement Book Series. Michigan State University
34. Pfaff MS, Drury JL, Klein GL (2015) Crowdsourcing mental models using DESIM (Descriptive to Executable Simulation Modeling). Presented at the international conference on natualistic decision making, McLean, VA
35. Giabbanelli PJ, Gray SA, Aminpour P (2017) Combining fuzzy cognitive maps with agent-based modeling: frameworks and pitfalls of a powerful hybrid modeling approach to understand human-environment interactions. Environ Model Softw 95:320–325
36. Zenobia B, Weber C, Daim T (2009) Artificial markets: a review and assessment of a new venue for innovation research. Technovation 29:338–350
37. Papageorgiou EI, Salmeron JL (2014) Methods and algorithms for fuzzy cognitive map-based modeling. Fuzzy cognitive maps for applied sciences and engineering. Springer, Berlin, Heidelberg, pp 1–28
38. Khoumbati K, Themistocleous M, Irani Z (2006) Evaluating the adoption of enterprise application integration in health-care organizations. J Manag Inf Syst 22:69–108
39. Spradley JP (1979) The ethnographic interview
40. Gray S, Chan A, Clark D, Jordan R (2012) Modeling the integration of stakeholder knowledge in social–ecological decision-making: benefits and limitations to knowledge diversity. Ecol Model 229:88–96
41. Anderson GO. Loneliness among older adults: a national survey of adults 45+. http://www.aarp.org/research/topics/life/info-2014/loneliness_2010.html

42. Liu L, Stroulia E, Nikolaidis I, Miguel-Cruz A, Rincon AR (2016) Smart homes and home health monitoring technologies for older adults: a systematic review. Int J Med Inf 91:44–59
43. O'Mara B, Gill GK, Babacan H, Donahoo D (2012) Digital technology, diabetes and culturally and linguistically diverse communities: a case study with elderly women from the Vietnamese community. Health Educ J 71:491–504

Part III
Machine Learning

Machine Learning for the Classification of Obesity from Dietary and Physical Activity Patterns

Arielle S. Selya and Drake Anshutz

Abstract Conventional epidemiological analyses in health-related research have been successful in identifying individual risk factors for adverse health outcomes, e.g. cigarettes' effect on lung cancer. However, for conditions that are multifactorial or for which multiple variables interact to affect risk, these approaches have been less successful. Machine learning approaches such as classifiers can improve risk prediction due to their ability to empirically detect *patterns* of variables that are "diagnostic" of a particular outcome, over the conventional approach of examining isolated, statistically independent relationships that are specified a priori. This chapter presents a proof-of-concept using several classifiers (discriminant analysis, support vector machines (SVM), and neural nets) to classify obesity from 18 dietary and physical activity variables. Random subsampling cross-validation was used to measure prediction accuracy. Classifiers outperformed logistic regressions: quadratic discriminant analysis (QDA) correctly classified 59% of cases versus logistic regression's 55% using original, unbalanced data; and radial-basis SVM classified nearly 61% of cases using balanced data, versus logistic regression's 59% prediction accuracy. Moreover, radial SVM predicted both categories (obese and non-obese) above chance simultaneously, while some other methods achieved above-chance prediction accuracy for only one category, usually to the detriment of the other. These findings show that obesity can be more accurately classified by a *combination* or *pattern* of dietary and physical activity behaviors, than by individual variables alone. Classifiers have the potential to inform more effective nutritional guidelines and treatments for obesity. More generally, machine learning methods can improve risk prediction for health outcomes over conventional epidemiological approaches.

A. S. Selya (✉) · D. Anshutz
Department of Population Health, University of North Dakota School
of Medicine & Health Sciences, Grand Forks, ND, USA
e-mail: arielle.selya@med.und.edu

© Springer International Publishing AG, part of Springer Nature 2018
P. J. Giabbanelli et al. (eds.), *Advanced Data Analytics in Health*, Smart Innovation, Systems and Technologies 93, https://doi.org/10.1007/978-3-319-77911-9_5

1 Introduction

Risk prediction of adverse health conditions and events is a primary goal of much medical and public health research. Typically, an early objective is identifying risk and/or protective factors for a given medical outcome based on regression-based analyses of data from some population of interest. Healthcare providers then use these risk factors to screen patients who are at risk in a broader population, and depending on the evidence for causality, can also use these risk factors as therapeutic targets. For example, high total serum cholesterol has been identified as a risk factor for cardiovascular disease (CVD) [1, 2], and patients are routinely prescribed statins in order to reduce their cholesterol and in turn their risk for cardiovascular disease [2]. Similarly, consuming a diet high in saturated fat is associated with obesity [3, 4], leading to recommendations to reduce dietary fat in order to reduce body weight [5].

1.1 Conventional Epidemiological Analyses: Technical Background

Conventional regression analyses (e.g. linear and logistic regressions) have led to great success in identifying risk factors and causes of some diseases, especially in cases where a single risk factor in isolation has a strong relationship with a medical outcome (e.g. establishing that cigarette smoking causes lung and other cancers). However, these approaches have made less progress in explaining other health outcomes, particularly multifactorial "lifestyle diseases" such as CVD, metabolic syndrome, and obesity. This is at least partly due to methodological limitations of these traditional approaches.

1.1.1 The Role of Parametric Assumptions

Conventional regressions make strong parametric assumptions about the relationships being examined in the data. In particular, regressions test for linear relationships between the predictor terms and the outcome. In the case of a linear regression, this means that each predictor is assumed to be linearly related to the outcome; and in the case of a logistic regression, to the log-odds of the outcome.

Violations of this linearity assumption can sometimes be corrected through pre-processing of variables such as logarithmic (e.g. as is done for age in predicting CVD [2]) or polynomial transformations. This allows certain types of nonlinearity, though the model tested is still linear in its relationship with the outcome. Additionally, a variable that is severely skewed or multimodal can be categorized, though this reduces the available information in the variable [6]. Thus, though these and other methods can to some extent alleviate the linearity assumption, they have important limitations.

Notably, regression analyses require the analyst to specify an equation in advance, and the regression analysis simply tests the data against this a priori hypothesis. Since the relationships that are actually tested in regression analyses are a small set of all possible relationships, this approach is likely to miss informative associations that are nonlinear.

1.1.2 Independent Terms Versus Interactions

In regression models, each predictor term (most commonly, a single variable) is examined after adjusting for the other terms in order to estimate statistically independent effects. Although this approach is valuable for isolating a single variable's effect among possible confounding influences, the interpretation of the corresponding findings is unclear when generalizing to real-world settings in which patterns of risk factors co-occur. This is the case with CVD: risk factors such as cigarette smoking, high blood pressure, and high cholesterol tend to correlate with each other, making the question of these factors' statistically independent contributions less meaningful and perhaps even a moot point. As a more extreme example, some claim that social status is the distal, underlying cause of such conditions [7].

In addition to examining statistically independent terms, regression models can also include interaction terms between two or more variables. Interactions or combinations of variables can be highly relevant for health research. For instance, consuming fish high in mercury is widely claimed to pose serious neurological risks [8], especially in utero [9]; however, more recent work shows that the selenium content of fish can nullify this risk [10]. That is, the *interaction* or *combination* of mercury and selenium is more important than knowing either factor in isolation.

However, regressions are limited in the extent to which they can examine patterns of variable interactions. Similar to the a priori specification of the shape of the regression equation (Sect. 1.1.1), particular interaction terms must also be specified in advance by the analyst. Specific interaction terms are typically motivated by previous literature and/or theory. For example, the 2013 American College of Cardiology (ACC)/American Heart Association (AHA) 10-year CVD risk prediction equations contain an interaction term between age and total cholesterol, and this is specifically included based on previous findings [2]. The need to justify interactions a priori means that it is not usually appropriate to exhaustively examine all possible interactions. This is especially true when examining simultaneous interactions: interaction terms add complexity to the model (especially terms with more than 2 interacting variables) and increase the required sample size. Thus, it is statistically infeasible to examine all possible interactions, which puts conventional regressions (e.g. linear and logistic regressions) at a disadvantage compared to the data-mining element of pattern-based classification analyses. Together, these limitations raise the possibility that unexamined interactions or patterns of variables could improve risk prediction. This limitation also applies to other related methods such as structural equation modeling (SEM), which model a set of regression equations simultaneously.

1.2 Machine Learning Approaches

Machine learning approaches offer an important complement to traditional regressions. Machine learning represents a broad array of different techniques, which can be broadly grouped based on whether learning is supervised (i.e., uses outcome data during training). Supervised methods include classifiers (the focus of this chapter), unsupervised methods include clustering, and semi-supervised methods include label propagation. A distinctive feature of classifiers is that they are empirically driven and have much fewer assumptions. First, classifiers are not always restricted to detecting linear information. Though some classifiers do have linear assumptions (e.g. that a linear decision surface can separate different classes), others do not and can thus detect complex, nonlinear relationships between variables.

Additionally, classifiers are better able to detect patterns of variables that are "diagnostic" of an outcome. As discussed in Sect. 1.1.2, regressions have a limited ability to examine interactions, but machine learning approaches can detect complex patterns without needing to specify them. Thus, classifiers have an exploratory, data mining element that is likely to uncover interaction effects that would have otherwise been missed by conventional linear or logistic regression analyses. Since these patterns can be combinatorial in nature (e.g. [11, 12]), it is informative not only what variables are "on" (i.e. have high values), but also which are "off" (i.e. have low values). As a result, pattern-based classification techniques are often superior at prediction due to the fact that *patterns* contain more information than the sum of independent variables alone.

1.2.1 Types of Classifiers

Three types of classifiers are presented here: discriminant analysis, support vector machines (SVM), and artificial neural nets (NN). All of these are supervised learning methods.

Bayesian classifiers create a decision surface that maximizes the difference between classes based on a combination of predictor variables; these are easily computed and do not require tuning of parameters. Two examples are linear discriminant analysis (LDA) which models a linear decision surface, and quadratic discriminant analysis (QDA) which models a quadratic surface [13].

SVM also models decision surfaces in the multivariate space of all predictor variables, by choosing a small number of "support vectors" that represent the most similar cases across classes (i.e. close to the decision surface that maximizes the difference between classes); remaining cases are classified based on which side of the support vectors they fall [14]. SVM is flexible with respect to parametric assumptions, and can be run with linear kernel or nonlinear (e.g. radial, polynomial, and sigmoid) kernels [14]. Parameters can be tuned for a better fit: cost to penalize misclassifications, and gamma to specify how far the influence of each training case reaches.

NN's map the predictor variables to an outcome variable through one or more intermediate "hidden layers" [15]. Each node (one per variable) in one layer is connected to each node in the next layer, and these connection weights are updated during training using the backpropogation algorithm, which results in the neural net "learning" an internal representation of the data and classification task [15, 16]. Parameter tuning is required to maximize the fit, such as the size of the hidden layer, number of training iterations, and weight decay.

1.2.2 Evaluation

Classifiers are evaluated in terms of how well they are able to separate classes of observations. Normally this evaluation involves some form of cross-validation testing, in which the available dataset is split into mutually exclusive "training" and "test" sets. The training set is used to train the classifier (e.g. establishing the decision surface), and the test set is used to examine generalization, i.e. how well the learned rules "predict" other cases. This method of cross-validation penalizes against overfitting and quantifies how well the classifier learned patterns that are truly diagnostic for a particular outcome class.

Cross-validation results can be presented in terms of confusion matrices, which for a binary classification task can be thought of in terms of hits, misses, false alarms, and correct rejections (Table 1). Overall prediction accuracy is an average of the correct classifications (i.e. correct rejections and hits). Other common metrics to evaluate classifiers can be derived from these, such as precision (the fraction of hits among all positively-classified cases) and recall (the fraction of hits among all actual positive cases).

The evaluation of classifiers differs substantially from the traditional evaluation of regressions. An important result of regression analyses is the significance testing ($p < 0.05$) of each predictor term, though it is essential to consider other aspects such as effect sizes [17, 18]. This approach can lead to identifying relationships that are statistically, but not *practically*, significant, especially when the sample size is large. For example, one study reported a significant relationship between dietary fat and obesity, but this was a difference of only 100 calories/day − less than 1/3rd of

Table 1 Structure of a confusion matrix for a binary prediction task

	Predicted class: 0	Predicted class: 1
Actual class: 0	Correct rejection	False alarm
Actual class: 1	Miss	Hit

the standard deviation in dietary fat consumption across the sample [19]. As a result, despite statistically significant differences *at the population level* for a certain risk factor, the variance is often so large that knowing *a particular individual's* measure has little to no predictive ability for their outcome (see Sect. 1.3). In such a situation, a model that fares well in a conventional regression analysis (i.e. identifying an association significant at $p < 0.05$) is likely to fare poorly if evaluated using prediction accuracy.

Regression models are also evaluated more globally by examining how well the model fits the data. For example, the R^2 statistic quantifies how much of the variance in the outcome variable is explained by the model (the shape of the equation and its set of predictor terms). Interpreting the R^2 when reporting on statistical testing can put into context the possible tension between statistical significance and practical significance; if the R^2 is very low, this indicates that the chosen set of predictors do not explain very much of the outcome, even if there is a small statistical association. Similarly, interpreting effect sizes, as is becoming increasingly required (e.g. [17]), can also guard against the shortfalls of significance testing.

1.3   Example: Predicting Obesity from Diet and Exercise Patterns

Obesity is a rising health problem in the United States, with over 30% of adults classified as obese [20]. Obesity poses a risk for many medical conditions, including type 2 diabetes and CVD [21]. Much existing research examines obesity from an energy balance perspective [22], postulating that it is caused by excess caloric consumption relative to metabolic energy expenditure. On the caloric intake side of the equation, individual components of one's diet have also been identified as risk factors for obesity. Dietary fat in particular has been implicated in higher body fat and obesity [19, 23], especially saturated fat [3].

However, this research suffers from the limitations discussed in Sect. 1.1, with the public health result that diet interventions and recommendations based on the assumed causal role of saturated fat have not been successful at actually reducing obesity [24]. One very relevant factor appears to be the type of calories used to replace the saturated fat in one's diet. For example, replacement with polyunsaturated fats seems to be beneficial in some respects, but not replacement with carbohydrates [24]. Alternatively, more recent research shows that low-carbohydrate diets can be at least as effective as low-fat diets for reducing body fat [24]. In other words, the *pattern* of macronutrients is more important than any single macronutrient. Finally, many of the reported associations between macronutrients and obesity are weak, despite being statistically significant (e.g. [19]), suggesting a low predictive ability of individual variables.

To illustrate the concept of prediction accuracy, consider the daily total fat consumption and its association with obesity among non-Hispanic white, female adults using real data from the National Health and Nutrition Examination Survey (NHANES), 2011 and 2013. To minimize the impact of energy expenditure, only those who reported no regular moderate or vigorous physical activity ($N = 892$) are considered.

On one hand, a hypothetical perfect prediction rule indicates that some cutoff value perfectly separates obese from non-obese individuals. At the other extreme, a completely unsuccessful prediction rule would mean obesity is randomly distributed with respect to caloric intake. The actual data (Fig. 1) look much closer to the hypothetical random case: although there is a trend for higher dietary fat intake among obese participants (127.6 g vs. 134.5 g, $p = 0.095$), there are a great many obese women with low fat intake, and many non-obese women with high fat intake. Though this difference did not reach statistical significance among this sample, a sample of all adults in NHANES showed that similar-magnitude differences did reach statistical significance (not presented) due to the increased sample size.

These existing difficulties in predicting and treating obesity make this topic a prime candidate for machine learning approaches. Some interesting work has already been published applying classifiers to study obesity. For example, random forests have identified social and geographical factors that are correlated with obesity [25]. Another study used decision trees to predict adherence to dietary recommendations [26]. Other work used machine learning to predict obesity from genetic data and childhood clinical factors [27, 28], microbiome data [29], and voice signals [30].

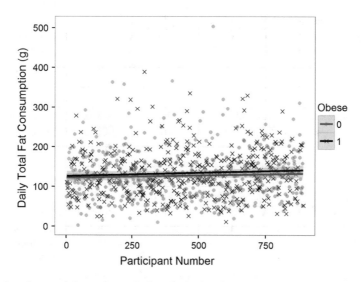

Fig. 1 Actual case of dietary fat predicting obesity in NHANES data

This chapter presents a proof-of-concept on the use of classifiers for predicting obesity status based on detailed information about diet and exercise. Data are drawn from NHANES, which contains detailed information from dietary interviews, physical examinations, and questionnaires. Three types of classifiers are used (discriminant analyses, SVM's, and NN's) to predict obesity status from diet, physical activity, and age. Prediction accuracy of each classifier and of a conventional logistic regression is calculated.

2   Methods

2.1   Sample

Data were drawn from NHANES, a large national survey of adults and children in the United States that is currently conducted biennially and is publicly available. NHANES has an extensive questionnaire component as well as a physical examination and laboratory component. In addition, a detailed dietary interview was conducted in which participants reported detailed food intake over the prior 24 h period. Data were obtained on each individual food/beverage, including the type of food in terms of the United States Department of Agriculture's (USDA's) Food Surveys Research Group (FSRP) categories, where the food was obtained, and the amount of food consumed in grams. This information was used to estimate the nutritional content of each meal and of each day. Data collection was performed using validated approaches developed by the USDA. Detailed data collection procedures are available in NHANES documentation [31]. Dietary information was assessed on two separate days. NHANES data and full documentation are publicly available online at https://www.cdc.gov/nchs/nhanes/index.htm.

Data from the 2011 and 2013 waves were pooled in order to increase sample size ($N = 19,931$). Participants under 21 ($N = 9033$) were excluded due to differing measures of obesity for youth. The main sample was further restricted to non-Hispanic, white females ($N = 2276$), which yielded the most accurate classification results in preliminary analyses. This was done because the classifiers used require quantitative, rather than categorical, predictor variables; thus a subgroup analysis is appropriate in order to account for group differences based on sex and race/ethnicity. Results using other groups in this NHANES data are briefly presented for comparison purposes following the main results.

Finally, all observations with missing data on any variables were removed, for a final sample size of $N = 2013$. Though there are a variety of ways to handle missing data, listwise deletion was used here as a conservative approach preserve the actual (and possibly nonlinear) patterns in the data and avoid distortion introduced by parametric assumptions (e.g. multiple imputation based on linear regression). Preliminary analyses (not presented) confirmed this concern in that multiple imputation of missing data disrupted some cases of successful classification.

2.2 Variables

The outcome variable of obesity was derived from body mass index (BMI) values from the physical examination component of NHANES, and was dichotomized based on the cutoff of 30 kg/m^2 [32].

Dietary variables totaled for each day included total energy in kilocalories (kcal), as well as the macronutrient content (protein, carbohydrate, and fat in grams). For the current study, these macronutrients were converted to fractions of total energy intake, using the conversions of 4 kcal/g for carbohydrate and protein and 9 kcal/g for fat. Components of these macronutrients were also used, including total sugars, saturated fatty acids, monounsaturated fatty acids, and polyunsaturated fatty acids (all in grams). Additionally, total dietary fiber (g), cholesterol (mg), alcohol (g), plain water (g), potassium (mg), and sodium (mg) were included in analyses. For participants who supplied two days of dietary interview, all variables were averaged across both days.

Three physical activity variables were derived from multiple items. First, physical inactivity was self-reported as the number of minutes per week the participant spends doing sedentary activities (e.g. watching television, using a computer). Second, moderate physical activity (minutes/week) was derived from questions assessing the number of days on which moderate physical activity is performed, and the number of minutes per day of moderate physical activity, both at work and for recreation. Additionally, the number of days and minutes per day spent walking or biking to work was also considered moderate physical activity as per NHANES' metabolic coding suggestions. The number of minutes was multiplied by the number of days, and the product was summed across settings (work, recreation, and walking/biking to work). Third, vigorous physical activity was derived similarly from responses about number of days and number of minutes/day spent on vigorous physical activity at work or for recreation.

Finally, age in years and height were included in analyses.

2.3 Analyses

The statistical software R [33] was used for all analyses. All predictor variables were normalized before analysis in order to equalize the signal across variables which differ in terms of units, scale, and variance. Considerations about normalized are discussed further in Sect. 4.4.1.

Since obese cases are rarer than non-obese cases, the dataset is considered to be unbalanced. This can negatively impact some classifiers, as the classification accuracy can reflect in part the proportion of each class. Therefore, a second dataset was constructed in order to balance the cases; this was done using the synthetic minority over-sampling technique (SMOTE), which generates new synthetic data points along a line between a data point and one of its nearest neighbors in feature space [34], implemented in the R package unbalanced [35]. The minority class (obese) was oversampled by 100%, and two majority class (non-obese) cases were sampled for each of these minority cases, resulting in a perfectly balanced dataset (50% of cases in each class). It is important to note that balancing is only performed on the training set, to prevent "learning" from exemplars based on the test set, which can artificially boost prediction accuracy. All analyses were run on both the original and balanced data.

Three types of classifiers were used to predict outcomes of obesity based on all predictor variables. First, discriminant analysis, both LDA and QDA, were performed using R's package MASS [36]. Second, SVM's were run with linear, radial, polynomial, and sigmoid kernels, using R's package e1071 [37]. Parameters of cost and gamma (for nonlinear kernels) were varied for optimization of prediction accuracy, each on an approximately logarithmic scale (cost values: 1, 3, 5, 10, 20, 50, 100; gamma: 0.01, 0.03, 0.05, 0.1, 0.2, 0.5, and 1). Finally, NN's were run using R's package nnet [36], and the size of the hidden layer (from 2 to 24 in increments of 2), the maximum number of iterations (from 100 to 400 in increments of 100), and the decay parameters (from 0 to 0.9 in increments of 0.1) were optimized.

Random subsampling cross-validation was used to evaluate the prediction accuracy of each classifier, each time holding out a random 10% of trials, with 1000 iterations each. Results were averaged across these 1000 iterations, which is necessary due to the large variation in results stemming from the random selection of the test set.

Cross-validation results were evaluated using confusion matrices (Sect. 1.2.2). Although classifier results are often presented in alternate formats such as precision, recall, and F1, the confusion matrix format is used here in order to more easily map the results to their clinical implications (e.g. optimal treatments/interventions would maximize the hit rate, while minimizing the miss rate and, if there are costs or side effects to the treatment/intervention, also minimizing the false alarm rate). Overall prediction accuracy was tested against chance using a binomial test of the success rate out of the 1000 iterations.

Finally, a logistic regression of obesity on all predictor variables was run. Though cross-validation is rarely used for logistic regressions, it was performed here for comparative purposes.

3   Results

Table 2 presents the confusion matrices from the best-case classifier, for both the original (unbalanced) data and the balanced data, along with any applicable parameters.

For the unbalanced data, QDA was the most accurate classifier, achieving a nearly 59% prediction accuracy. By comparison, the logistic regression achieved only a 55% prediction accuracy, though this was significantly above chance.

Table 2 Prediction (test set) confusion matrices of each classifier, using the original, unbalanced data (top sub-row) and the balanced data (bottom sub-row)

Type of classifier	Instance	Dataset (parameters)		Not obese	obese
Bayesian	LDA	Original	Not obese (%)	**86.9**	13.1
			Obese (%)	77.4	**22.6**
			Average (%)	**54.8**	
		Balanced	Not obese (%)	**53.7**	46.3
			Obese (%)	35.2	**64.8**
			Average (%)	**59.0**	
	QDA	Original	Not obese (%)	**62.7**	37.3
			Obese (%)	45.3	**54.7**
			Average (%)	**58.7**	
		Balanced	Not obese (%)	**38.7**	61.3
			Obese (%)	20.8	**79.2**
			Average (%)	**58.9**	
SVM	Linear	Original (cost = 1)	Not obese (%)	100	0
			Obese (%)	100	0
			Average (%)	**50**	
		Balanced (cost = 10)	Not obese (%)	**48.9**	51.1
			Obese (%)	30.0	**70.0**
			Average (%)	**59.5**	
	Radial	Original (cost = 10, gamma = 0.1)	Not obese (%)	**71.5**	28.5
			Obese (%)	57.1	**42.9**
			Average (%)	**57.2**	
		Balanced (cost = 3, gamma = 0.03)	Not obese	**58.1**	41.9
			Obese (%)	36.7	**63.2**
			Average (%)	**60.7**	
	Polynomial	Original (cost = 100, gamma = 0.05)	Not obese (%)	**72.6**	27.4
			Obese (%)	62.1	**37.9**
			Average (%)	**55.2**	
		Balanced (cost = 100, gamma = 0.05)	Not obese (%)	**50.1**	49.9
			Obese (%)	40.1	**59.9**
			Average (%)	**55.0**	
	Sigmoid	Original (cost = 10, gamma = 0.5)	Not obese (%)	42.8	47.2
			Obese (%)	44.0	60.0
			Average (%)	49.4	
		Balanced (cost = 10, gamma = 0.01)	Not obese (%)	**52.1**	47.9
			Obese (%)	43.3	**56.6**
			Average (%)	**54.4**	

(continued)

Table 2 (continued)

Type of classifier	Instance	Dataset (parameters)		Not obese	obese
NN		Original (size = 6, max. iter. = 200, decay = 0.1)	Not obese (%)	**73.5**	26.5
			Obese (%)	58.3	**41.7**
			Average (%)	**57.6**	
		Balanced (size = 8, max. iter. = 200, decay = 0.3)	Not obese (%)	**57.3**	42.7
			Obese (%)	42.1	**57.9**
			Average (%)	**57.6**	
Logistic regression		Original	Not obese (%)	**86.0**	14.0
			Obese (%)	75.4	**24.6**
			Average (%)	**55.3**	
		Balanced	Not obese (%)	**54.0**	46.0
			Obese (%)	35.6	**64.4**
			Average (%)	**59.2**	

Note LDA Linear discriminant analysis. *QDA* Quadratic discriminant analysis. *SVM* Support vector machines. *NN* Neural net. Size Number of nodes in the hidden layer. *Max. iter.* Maximum number of iterations
Bold: Averaged prediction accuracy across the two classes is statistically different chance, based on a binomial test of the success rate out of 1000 trials

Additionally, only QDA was able to separate the two classes successfully, based on the above-chance classifications for both categories simultaneously. In contrast, logistic regression and all other classifiers showed a bias towards "not obese:" though they correctly identified those who were not obese with a high degree of accuracy, this was at the expense of a high miss rate. Thus, despite the above-chance prediction accuracies in most cases, these are considered unsuccessful classifications due to the below-chance classification accuracy for "obese." This bias in these classifiers reflects the imbalance in the data set, i.e. the higher prevalence of "not obese" cases.

Prediction accuracy was generally higher using the balanced dataset. In particular, radial SVM's achieved the highest prediction accuracy at 60.7%. Using a balanced dataset also improved the accuracy of the logistic regression to 59.2%, which was on par with LDA at 59.0%. Thus, in this case, balancing the dataset narrowed the advantage of the classifiers relative to logistic regression. Other classifiers also showed bias, this time towards "obese," though the magnitude of the bias often decreased after balancing.

Regarding parameter tuning, SVM did not consistently show higher prediction accuracies with any specific cost and gamma values. That is, different combinations of these parameters may influence one SVM model differently than another one. Evaluating all parameter combinations within each SVM model is crucial for thoroughly optimizing prediction accuracy.

Similar results were obtained when analyzing other groups within the NHANES sample, with nonlinear SVM's matching or exceeding the performance of logistic regressions. Among white males, no method was able to successfully classify both classes in the original above chance, but QDA had a small but reliable improvement rate over logistic regression (56.7% vs. 55.9%) when classifying the balanced data. Among Hispanic females, radial SVM correctly classified 53.0% of cases which was a slight improvement over the logistic regression's 52.4% average prediction accuracy.

4 Discussion

4.1 Summary

This chapter presents a proof-of-concept of using cross-validated classifiers, a type of machine learning analysis, to predict obesity status from a wide range of diet and physical activity variables using national survey data. QDA was most successful at classifying the original (imbalanced) dataset, achieving nearly a 60% average prediction accuracy; an improvement of nearly 4% over logistic regression. For the balanced data, radial SVM was most successful at nearly 61% average prediction accuracy. This remained reliably more accurate than logistic regression, although balancing the data reduced classifiers' relative improvement. Other classifiers were unsuccessful, often showing a bias towards one category, at the expense of the other. However, balancing allowed more classifiers to successfully classify both categories above chance simultaneously. Together, these results demonstrate that classifiers can reliably increase the risk prediction of health outcomes versus conventional regressions.

The current demonstration that classifiers can improve risk prediction or classification corroborates previous research on a wide range of health topics. Classifiers have been previously used to predict obesity [25, 27–30, 38] and compliance with dietary recommendations [26], and to improve detection of different types of physical activity [39]. Classifiers have also been successfully applied to other fields, including predicting metabolic syndrome from physical characteristics and laboratory results [40], identifying binge drinkers from parenting variables [41] and drinking motives [42], predicting high blood pressure using body measures [43], examining differences in smoking behavior and nicotine dependence across subpopulations of smokers [44, 45], and predicting patterns of neurophysiological activity that underlie object categorization in the visual cortex [11, 12].

4.2 Implications for Health

A majority of existing research on dietary determinants of obesity focuses on statistically independent associations of individual dietary variables with outcomes of obesity. Unfortunately, this existing body of research has not yet been successful in identifying a simple and effective solution [24].

The ability of the best-case classifier to predict obesity more accurately based on diet and exercise patterns, relative to conventional logistic regression, has wide-ranging implications for understanding, preventing, and reducing obesity. First, these findings confirm relatively recent research suggesting that combinations of dietary components have explanatory power for obesity that is higher than what can be achieved with the sum of the individual components. The importance of *patterns* of dietary components also offers an explanation for difficulties plaguing much existing research on nutritional determinants of obesity: that there is inconsistent evidence for the link between any single macronutrient and obesity [24]; and that even when significant, the effects are weak (e.g. [19]) and thus provide little-to-no predictive power for a given individual. The conflicting evidence in this body of research has produced dietary guidelines that, in some cases, do not fully reflect the research on the role of diet in CVD risk [46] and that have been retracted over time (e.g. limits on dietary cholesterol [5]).

These classifiers can be used to predict new cases based on dietary and physical activity patterns. It is appropriate to test different types of classifiers with different decision surfaces to find the best fit for the data. Once the model is optimized and trained, it could conceivably be used to predict an individual's risk of obesity. The ease of collecting data must also be taken into account; it is much easier to directly measure obesity in healthcare settings than to collect detailed dietary information. However, in real-world settings, and with the preponderance of smartphones and apps that estimate nutritional information from image files and calories burned during exercise, there could be substantial clinical value in predicting the risk of obesity based on real-world dietary and physical activity patterns and flagging "risky" behaviors. In fact, such devices have been and continue to be researched and developed. Wearable devices such as accelerometers and/or barometers, along with machine learning approaches, can accurately measure and classify different types of physical activity [39, 47] and estimate energy expenditure [48, 49]. Additionally, a variety of portable, wearable and implanted devices can estimate dietary intake via acoustic monitoring, images of food, or motion detection of chewing and swallowing [for a review, see 50].

Additionally, the current findings could be built upon by analyzing the results of this QDA model to determine which variables contribute most to the classification task (see Sect. 4.4.2), though this may fail to capture some important "diagnostic" information contained in interactions or patterns (see Sect. 4.3.2). Such an analysis would identify sets of variables that are correlated (positively or negatively) with obesity. The next stage would randomized experiments based on these sets of dietary patterns to test whether they represent *causal* relationships that either increase the risk of obesity or protect against it. If these findings are validated in other samples and using such data from randomized experiments to establish causality, they could be used to inform more effective dietary guidelines in the future.

Finally, a cost-benefit analyses based in part on the current findings could estimate the potential savings from the increased prediction accuracy afforded by classifiers. Better prediction would result in more patients at risk receiving the treatment or intervention they need. Additionally factoring in data on the per-person costs of obesity and the success rate of intervention or treatment would yield the cost savings of correctly treating patients who are "hits." The false alarm rate is also essential to consider, as this translates into the possible costs and harms of unnecessarily treating these patients. For example, aggressive prostate cancer screening has led to a great deal of over-diagnosis and unnecessary treatment in men who are likely to never have developed clinical symptoms [51], which high-lights the importance of a low false-alarm rate when considering costs and benefits.

4.3 Other Considerations When Using Classifiers Versus Regressions

4.3.1 Data Considerations

Many machine learning approaches are limited in terms of types of variables (e.g. continuous or categorical). In particular, the classifiers presented here require numeric variables. However, categorical variables such as age and race/ethnicity are strongly associated with virtually all other health outcomes.

Therefore, one advantage of regression analyses over the classifiers used here is that they can handle both continuous and categorical variables simultaneously, and thus use a greater *number* of predictor variables. This could in theory boost the prediction accuracy above that of classifiers that are restricted to the subset of numeric variables. It is worth noting that this was not true in the current example based on follow-up analyses (not presented): using the full sample of adults (both sexes and all race/ethnicity values), the best-case classifier still outperformed logistic regression to a similar degree as above (Sect. 3) in terms of both classifi-cation accuracy and the ability to successfully separate the classes, despite the inclusion of additional variables (sex and race/ethnicity) in the logistic regression.

One way to account for categorical differences in machine learning is to split the set of observations into subgroups based on the categorical variable of interest (or intersections of more than one categorical variable) and run classifiers separately within each subgroup. Such an analysis could identify different patterns of variables that are predictive for each subgroup. This type of subgroup analysis is also commonly used in conventional epidemiological analyses: for example, the 2013 ACC/AHA 10 year CVD risk calculator has differing sets of predictor variables for each subset of race and sex [2]. Thus, this limitation of classifiers relative to conventional regressions can be small and/or manageable.

Additionally, other types of classifiers not presented here can use categorical variables, such as decision trees and association rules. Such classifiers would be a more appropriate choice if the available data contains several categorical variables that are thought to be important; and of course, continuous variables could be categorized in this case (e.g. based on clinical cutoff values) in order to increase the number of available variables for prediction.

The type of outcome variable also determines which methods are appropriate. The classifiers used here require categorical outcome variables. The current analyses present a binary classification task; however, these same classifiers could also perform a multilevel classification task (e.g. normal weight vs. overweight vs. obese). This is typically handled as a series of pairwise binary classification tasks; the methods used here automatically integrate these so that there are no additional steps required of the user compared to a simple binary classification task.

On the other hand, for continuous outcome variables, other types of machine learning (e.g. SVM regression) are available. An SVM regression would be appropriate, for example, if numeric BMI instead of binary BMI was used as the outcome. Similarly, different types of regressions are used for different types of outcomes (e.g. linear regression for continuous outcomes and logistic for binary outcomes).

Sample size is another important consideration. A rough guideline for regressions is that 10–20 observations are necessary per independent variable [6], though the sample size requirements for a given effect size and model can be determined more specifically by power analyses [18]. The required sample size for classifiers is not straightforward. Typically, classifiers are used on large samples, though in some cases have been used on as few as ≈ 100 observations per class for testing and training [52]. For either method, it is possible to use bootstrapping (i.e. repeated sampling from the original pool of observations with replacement) in order to increase precision of effect estimates with small sample sizes.

4.3.2 Interpretability of Results

Another major disadvantage of some pattern-based machine learning approaches is interpretability of the findings with respect to which variables are most informative for the classification task. That is, since there is often substantial information contained in *patterns* of variables, it is difficult (and not always sensible or useful) to quantify the role of individual variables. The classifiers used in this study are "black boxes" to an extent, and trade off interpretability for their primary advantage of detecting pattern-based "diagnostic" information. This is at odds with the tendency of healthcare professionals towards simple rules that identify a single variable which can act both as a risk indicator and therapeutic target.

However, other classifiers not examined here which produce more easily interpretable results. For example, decision trees or rule sets are much more transparent and interpretable. These types of classifiers may be more appropriate for research questions in which the need for interpretability is high; whereas "black-box" classifiers (e.g. SVM) may be more appropriate if classification accuracy is more important.

One solution to the trade-off between interpretability and increased predictive accuracy is to separate the *risk prediction* on one hand from the *intervention or treatment* on the other hand. It is possible that the signal is different from the cause, or that the most effective treatment is different from the signal. For example, though dietary and exercise patterns are clearly a *signal* for obesity, their causal impact remains inconclusive [24]. Instead, unrelated variables such as sleep duration [53] or cumulative antibiotic use [54] may be stronger *causes* of obesity and could possibly serve as more effective intervention targets.

4.4 Other Analytical Options

4.4.1 Data Preprocessing

In this example, all variables were normalized prior to classification. This has the effect of putting all variables on the same scale, so that nutrients consumed in larger quantities and/or with greater variance do not overwhelm the signals of nutrients contained in smaller amounts. However, that type of "weighting" might be desirable depending on the data and research question. That is, the original, unscaled variables may be more informative in cases when the large-magnitude variables carry more information than lower-magnitude and/or more stable variables. Since this is not often known a priori, it is reasonable to run preliminary tests using both standardized and unstandardized variables.

Other preprocessing methods to reduce dimensionality can also be effective, especially for high-dimensional data. Useful methods include principal components analysis (PCA), multidimensional scaling (MDS), or clustering analysis. These methods can reduce the number of dimensions necessary to represent the variation in the data. For example, if using PCA, one could use enough principal components to capture 95% of the variance in the original data; and if using MDS, enough variables to achieve *stress* < 5. The new transformed variables can then be used as predictors in the classifiers. It is important to note that the outcome variable should not be included in the dataset when performing these methods; this would artificially inflate the true classification accuracy. In the current example, using PCA or MDS for dimensionality reduction did not improve the classification accuracy (not presented).

4.4.2 Model Analysis

After optimizing and training a successful classifier, the researcher often desires to determine the most important variables for the classification task. This can be done in different ways depending on the type of classifier (see [11, 12]). However, classifier-specific methods make it difficult to compare results across different types of classifiers. A valuable alternative is sensitivity analysis, in which Gaussian noise of fixed magnitude is added to each variable, averaged over many iterations, to determine its effect on prediction accuracy. Noise added to variables that are important to the classification task will disrupt the prediction accuracy to a larger degree than it will when added to less important variables, and a threshold of change in prediction accuracy can be used to identify the most salient variables (e.g. [12]). However, any of these model analyses should be interpreted with caution, as "forcing" the question of which individual variables are important is likely to overlook important patterns (see Sect. 4.3.2).

4.5   Limitations

The current findings are limited due to the nature of the data (see Sect. 4.3 for methodological limitations). First, the data are observational and cannot be used to establish causal relationships. The accuracy of dietary variables are limited by self-report and recall; however, the validated data collection procedures [31] minimize these errors. The current sample analysis does not account for weight loss attempts, special diets, or the quantity of food consumed during interview days compared with usual intake. This likely has the effect of making the classification more difficult due to increased variance, but does not otherwise invalidate the results. As a result, these findings reflect conservative estimates of prediction accuracies, and further subgroup analyses may be warranted in future research based on such variables. Finally, the current analysis does not incorporate NHANES' survey weights, and these specific findings may not generalize to larger populations. However, the primary goal of this chapter is to provide a proof-of-concept that machine learning analyses can outperform conventional regression analyses in the prediction of health outcomes. Additional research is needed to confirm the substantive contribution of this work to obesity research, ideally using objectively-measured data and randomized study designs.

4.6   Conclusions

This chapter demonstrates that classifiers achieved a higher prediction accuracy than conventional logistic regression in predicting obesity from dietary and physical activity variables. This finding demonstrates that *patterns* of dietary and exercise behavior, rather than individual components, can better explain the prevalence of obesity. Additional research into specific patterns of dietary intake are warranted to inform more effective nutritional guidelines in the future. More generally, this work serves as a proof-of-concept that machine learning analyses can substantially improve upon conventional epidemiological approaches to risk prediction of health outcomes.

References

1. Kannel WB, Dawber TR, Kagan A, Revotskie N, Stokes J III (1961) Factors of risk in the development of coronary heart disease–six year follow-up experience. The Framingham study. Ann Intern Med 55:33–50

2. Goff DJ, Lloyd-Jones D, Bennett G, Coady S, D'Agostino RBS, Gibbons R, Greenland P, Lackland D, Levy D, O'Donnell CRJ, Schwartz J, Smith SJ, Sorlie P, Shero S, Stone N, WIlson P (2014) 2013 ACC/AHA guideline on the assessment of cardiovascular risk: a report of the American College of Cardiology/American Heart Association Task Force on practice guidelines. Circulation 129(suppl 2):S49–S73. https://doi.org/10.1161/01.cir.0000437741.48606.98

3. Crescenzo R, Bianco F, Mazzoli A, Giacco A, Cancelliere R, di Fabio G, Zarrelli A, Liverini G, Iossa S (2015) Fat quality influences the obesogenic effect of high fat diets. Nutrients 7(11):9475–9491. https://doi.org/10.3390/nu7115480

4. Riccardi G, Giacco R, Rivellese AA (2004) Dietary fat, insulin sensitivity and the metabolic syndrome. Clin Nutr 23(4):447–456. https://doi.org/10.1016/j.clnu.2004.02.006

5. U.S. Department of Health and Human Services, U.S. Department of Agriculture (2015) 2015–2020 dietary guidelines for Americans, 8th edn

6. Harrell F (2015) Regression modeling strategies: with applications to linear models, logistic and ordinal regression, and survival analysis. In: Springer series in statistics. Springer

7. Link BG, Phelan J (1995) Social conditions as fundamental causes of disease. J Health Soc Behav 80–94

8. Carocci A, Rovito N, Sinicropi MS, Genchi G (2014) Mercury toxicity and neurodegenerative effects. Rev Environ Contam Toxicol 229:1–18. https://doi.org/10.1007/978-3-319-03777-6_1

9. Solan TD, Lindow SW (2014) Mercury exposure in pregnancy: a review. J Perinat Med 42 (6):725–729. https://doi.org/10.1515/jpm-2013-0349

10. Ralston NV, Ralston CR, Raymond LJ (2016) Selenium health benefit values: updated criteria for mercury risk assessments. Biol Trace Elem Res 171(2):262–269. https://doi.org/10.1007/s12011-015-0516-z

11. Hanson SJ, Schmidt A (2011) High-resolution imaging of the fusiform face area (FFA) using multivariate non-linear classifiers shows diagnosticity for non-face categories. Neuroimage 54 (2):1715–1734. https://doi.org/10.1016/j.neuroimage.2010.08.028

12. Hanson SJ, Matsuka T, Haxby JV (2004) Combinatorial codes in ventral temporal lobe for object recognition: Haxby (2001) revisited: is there a "face" area? Neuroimage 23(1):156–166. https://doi.org/10.1016/j.neuroimage.2004.05.020

13. Duda RO, Hart PE, Stork DG (2000) Pattern classification. Wiley, New York

14. Cristianini N, Shawe-Taylor J (2000) An introduction to support vector machines and other Kernel-based learning methods. Cambridge University Press, Cambridge, UK

15. Rumelhart DE, McClelland JL (1986) Psychological and biological models. MIT Press, Cambridge, MA

16. Rumelhart DE, Hinton GE, Williams RJ (1986) Learning representations by back-propagating errors. Nature 323(6088):533–536

17. American Psychological Association (2010) Publication manual of the American Psychological Association, 6th edn. American Psychological Association, Washington, D.C

18. Cohen J (1988) Statistical power analysis for the behavioral sciences, 2 edn. Lawrence Erlbaum Associates

19. Satia-Abouta J, Patterson RE, Schiller RN, Kristal AR (2002) Energy from fat is associated with obesity in U.S. men: results from the prostate cancer prevention Trial. Prev Med 34 (5):493–501. https://doi.org/10.1006/pmed.2002.1018

20. Ogden CL, Carroll MD, Fryar CD, Flegal KM (2015) Prevalence of obesity among adults and youth: United States, 2011–2014. NCHS data brief, vol 219, Hyattsville, MD

21. National Institutes of Health (1998) Clinical guidelines on the identification, evaluation, and treatment of overweight and obesity in adults. vol NIH Publication No. 98-4083. U.S. Department of Health and Human Services, Public Health Service, National Institutes of Health, and National Heart, Lung, and Blood Institute
22. Hill JO, Wyatt HR, Peters JC (2012) Energy balance and obesity. Circulation 126(1):126–132. https://doi.org/10.1161/circulationaha.111.087213
23. Tucker LA, Kano MJ (1992) Dietary fat and body fat: a multivariate study of 205 adult females. Am J Clin Nutr 56(4):616–622
24. Walker TB, Parker MJ (2014) Lessons from the war on dietary fat. J Am Coll Nutr 33(4):347–351. https://doi.org/10.1080/07315724.2013.870055
25. Nau C, Ellis H, Huang H, Schwartz BS, Hirsch A, Bailey-Davis L, Kress AM, Pollak J, Glass TA (2015) Exploring the forest instead of the trees: an innovative method for defining obesogenic and obesoprotective environments. Health Place 35:136–146. https://doi.org/10.1016/j.healthplace.2015.08.002
26. Giabbanelli PJ, Adams J (2016) Identifying small groups of foods that can predict achievement of key dietary recommendations: data mining of the UK National Diet and Nutrition survey, 2008–12. Public Health Nutr 19(9):1543–1551. https://doi.org/10.1017/S1368980016000185
27. Seyednasrollah F, Makela J, Pitkanen N, Juonala M, Hutri-Kahonen N, Lehtimaki T, Viikari J, Kelly T, Li C, Bazzano L, Elo LL, Raitakari OT (2017) Prediction of adulthood obesity using genetic and childhood clinical risk factors in the cardiovascular risk in Young Finns study. Circ Cardiovasc Genet 10(3). https://doi.org/10.1161/circgenetics.116.001554
28. Dugan TM, Mukhopadhyay S, Carroll A, Downs S (2015) Machine learning techniques for prediction of early childhood obesity. Appl Clin Inform 6(3):506–520. https://doi.org/10.4338/aci-2015-03-ra-0036
29. Sze MA, Schloss PD (2016) Looking for a signal in the noise: revisiting obesity and the microbiome. mBio 7(4). https://doi.org/10.1128/mbio.01018-16
30. Lee BJ, Kim KH, Ku B, Jang JS, Kim JY (2013) Prediction of body mass index status from voice signals based on machine learning for automated medical applications. Artif Intell Med 58(1):51–61. https://doi.org/10.1016/j.artmed.2013.02.001
31. Centers for Disease Control and Prevention, National Center for Health Statistics (2014) National Health and Nutrition Examination Survey (NHANES) MEC In-Person Dietary Interviewers Procedures Manual. Centers for Disease Control and Prevention
32. Centers for Disease Control and Prevention (2016) Defining adult overweight and obesity. Centers for Disease Control and Prevention. https://www.cdc.gov/obesity/adult/defining.html. Accessed 21 June 2017
33. Team RC (2016) R: a language and environment for statistical computing. R Foundation for Statistical Computing, Vienna, Austria
34. Chawla NV, Bowyer KW, Hall LO, Kegelmeyer WP (2002) SMOTE: synthetic minority over-sampling technique. J Artif Intell Res 16:321–357
35. Dal Pazzolo A, Caelen O, Bontempi G (2015) Unbalanced: racing for unbalanced methods selection. R package version, 2.0 edn
36. Venables WN, Ripley BD (2002) Modern applied statistics with S, 4th edn. Springer, New York
37. Meyer D, Dimitriadou E, Hornik K, Weingessel A, Leisch F (2015) e1071: misc functions of the department of statistics. R package version 1.6-7 edn. Probability Theory Group (Formerly: E1071), TU Wien
38. Thaiss CA, Itav S, Rothschild D, Meijer M, Levy M, Moresi C, Dohnalova L, Braverman S, Rozin S, Malitsky S, Dori-Bachash M, Kuperman Y, Biton I, Gertler A, Harmelin A, Shapiro H, Halpern Z, Aharoni A, Segal E, Elinav E (2016) Persistent microbiome alterations modulate the rate of post-dieting weight regain. Nature. https://doi.org/10.1038/nature20796
39. Kerr J, Patterson RE, Ellis K, Godbole S, Johnson E, Lanckriet G, Staudenmayer J (2016) Objective assessment of physical activity: classifiers for public health. Med Sci Sports Exerc 48(5):951–957. https://doi.org/10.1249/mss.0000000000000841

40. Karimi-Alavijeh F, Jalili S, Sadeghi M (2016) Predicting metabolic syndrome using decision tree and support vector machine methods. ARYA Atherosclerosis 12(3):146–152
41. Crutzen R, Giabbanelli PJ, Jander A, Mercken L, de Vries H (2015) Identifying binge drinkers based on parenting dimensions and alcohol-specific parenting practices: building classifiers on adolescent-parent paired data. BMC Public Health 15:747. https://doi.org/10.1186/s12889-015-2092-8
42. Crutzen R, Giabbanelli P (2014) Using classifiers to identify binge drinkers based on drinking motives. Subst Use Misuse 49(1–2):110–115
43. Golino HF, Amaral LS, Duarte SF, Gomes CM, Soares Tde J, Dos Reis LA, Santos J (2014) Predicting increased blood pressure using machine learning. J Obes 2014:637635. https://doi.org/10.1155/2014/637635
44. Dierker L, Rose J, Tan X, Li R (2010) Uncovering multiple pathways to substance use: a comparison of methods for identifying population subgroups. J Prim Prev 31(5–6):333–348. https://doi.org/10.1007/s10935-010-0224-6
45. Pugach O, Cannon DS, Weiss RB, Hedeker D, Mermelstein RJ (2017) Classification tree analysis as a method for uncovering relations between CHRNA5A3B4 and CHRNB3A6 in predicting smoking progression in adolescent smokers. Nicotine Tob Res 19(4):410–416. https://doi.org/10.1093/ntr/ntw197
46. Hoenselaar R (2012) Saturated fat and cardiovascular disease: the discrepancy between the scientific literature and dietary advice. Nutrition (Burbank, Los Angeles County, Calif) 28(2):118–123. https://doi.org/10.1016/j.nut.2011.08.017
47. Boateng G, Batsis JA, Halter R, Kotz D (2017) ActivityAware: an app for real-time daily activity level monitoring on the amulet wrist-worn device. In: Proceedings of the IEEE international conference on pervasive computing and communications workshops 2017. https://doi.org/10.1109/percomw.2017.7917601
48. Pande A, Zhu J, Das AK, Zeng Y, Mohapatra P, Han JJ (2015) Using smartphone sensors for improving energy expenditure estimation. IEEE J Transl Eng Health Med 3:2700212. https://doi.org/10.1109/jtehm.2015.2480082
49. Taylor D, Murphy J, Ahmad M, Purkayastha S, Scholtz S, Ramezani R, Vlaev I, Blakemore AI, Darzi A (2016) Quantified-self for obesity: physical activity behaviour sensing to improve health outcomes. Stud Health Technol Inform 220:414–416
50. Prioleau T, Moore E, Ghovanloo M (2017) Unobtrusive and wearable systems for automatic dietary monitoring. IEEE Trans Biomed Eng 99:1–1. https://doi.org/10.1109/tbme.2016.2631246
51. Tabayoyong W, Abouassaly R (2015) Prostate cancer screening and the associated controversy. Surg Clin N Am 95(5):1023–1039. https://doi.org/10.1016/j.suc.2015.05.001
52. Beleites C, Neugebauer U, Bocklitz T, Krafft C, Popp J (2013) Sample size planning for classification models. Anal Chim Acta 760:25–33. https://doi.org/10.1016/j.aca.2012.11.007
53. Beccuti G, Pannain S (2011) Sleep and obesity. Curr Opin Clin Nutr Metab Care 14(4):402–412. https://doi.org/10.1097/MCO.0b013e3283479109
54. Turta O, Rautava S (2016) Antibiotics, obesity and the link to microbes—what are we doing to our children? BMC Med 14:57. https://doi.org/10.1186/s12916-016-0605-7

Classifying Mammography Images by Using Fuzzy Cognitive Maps and a New Segmentation Algorithm

Abdollah Amirkhani, Mojtaba Kolahdoozi, Elpiniki I. Papageorgiou and Mohammad R. Mosavi

Abstract Mammography is one of the best techniques for the early detection of breast cancer. In this chapter, a method based on fuzzy cognitive map (FCM) and its evolutionary-based learning capabilities is presented for classifying mammography images. The main contribution of this work is two-fold: (a) to propose a new segmentation approach called the threshold based region growing (TBRG) algorithm for segmentation of mammography images, and (b) to implement FCM method in the context of mammography image classification by developing a new FCM learning algorithm efficient for tumor classification. By applying the proposed (TBRG) algorithm, a possible tumor is delineated against the background tissue. We extracted 36 features from the tissue, describing the texture and the boundary of the segmented region. Due to the curse of dimensionality of features space, the features were selected with the help of the continuous particle swarm optimization algorithm. The FCM was trained using a new evolutionary approach based on the area under curve (AUC) of the output concept. In order to evaluate the efficacy of the presented scheme, comparisons with benchmark machine learning algorithms were conducted and known metrics like ROC, AUC were calculated. The AUC obtained for the test data set is 87.11%, which indicates the excellent performance of the proposed FCM.

A. Amirkhani (✉) · M. Kolahdoozi · M. R. Mosavi
Department of Electrical Engineering, Iran University of Science and Technology,
16846-13114 Tehran, Iran
e-mail: amirkhani@ieee.org; amiramirkhani67@gmail.com

M. Kolahdoozi
e-mail: mojtaba_kolahdoozi@elec.iust.ac.ir

E. I. Papageorgiou
Computer Engineering Department, Technological Educational Institute
of Central Greece, Lamia, Greece

E. I. Papageorgiou
Department of Computer Science, University of Thessaly, 35100 Lamia, Greece

© Springer International Publishing AG, part of Springer Nature 2018
P. J. Giabbanelli et al. (eds.), *Advanced Data Analytics in Health*, Smart Innovation,
Systems and Technologies 93, https://doi.org/10.1007/978-3-319-77911-9_6

Keywords Fuzzy cognitive map · Mammography images · Breast tumor
Region growing

1 Introduction

Breast cancer is one of the most deadly cancers among women. The mortality rate
of breast cancer in the USA is higher than that of any other cancer type [1].
Although breast cancer is potentially a deadly disease, its early detection can
substantially help and alleviate the treatment process and increase the survival rate
of patients.

Although mammography is one of the most effective tools for the early diagnosis
of breast cancer, a study in Japan [2] revealed that about 23% of cancers cases are
not diagnosed, through mammography, by radiologists. Also another research [3]
demonstrates that about 17% of cancers are not diagnosed in U.S. using mammography images. This calls for the development of novel methods for breast
cancer detection.

In this chapter, an automatic method is presented for classifying mammography
images into benign or cancerous ones. First, the images are preprocessed in order to
eliminate extraneous factors such as noise or unwanted labels. Then by using a new
segmentation algorithm (called threshold based region growing (TBRG)), which
belongs to the family of region growing algorithms, the acquired mammography
images are segmented. After segmenting the images, 36 features are extracted for
the purpose of describing the texture and the boundaries of segmented regions. In
the next step, the desired features are selected by using the particle swarm optimization (PSO) algorithm [4, 5]. Finally, the features selected in the previous step
are classified through fuzzy cognitive map (FCM).

Main contributions of our work can be summarized as follow:

1. Proposing a new region growing algorithm called 'TBRG' for segmentation of
   mammography images.
2. Implementing FCMs for the first time in the context of mammography image
   classification by developing a new FCM learning algorithm efficient for
   classification.

The remainder of this chapter has been organized as follows: Sect. 2 reviews
previous works on the mammography images classification. Section 3 describes the
proposed algorithm for classification of mammography images. Section 4 contains
the empirical results obtained by applying the FCM algorithm on the digital
database for screening mammography (DDSM) dataset. And finally, the conclusion
of this research is presented in Sect. 5.

2 Background

Medical image analysis could help the experts to raise the accuracy in diagnosing several diseases. Despite major advances in mammography image processing, there are still many challenges: the automatic segmentation of mammography images as accurate as radiologists [6], processing images of dense breasts as accurately as processing the images of normal breasts [7], implementing a method similar to the human reasoning method to reach higher levels of accuracy [8], and finding dedicated mammography image descriptors capable of high interclass and low dimensional resolution [9]. Due to recent research achievements and modern technology, researchers have investigated certain approaches, aiming to reach accuracy levels above 85% in classification [10], accomplish mammography image segmentation with the Jaccard index above 70% [11], enhance clarity and remove noise from mammography images [12], and develop preprocessing methods preventing significant differences in extracted features [13].

This section deals with some of the most important studies conducted in this field.

Breast cancers can be visualized in mammography images in two forms which are microcalcifications and massive lesions. It is difficult to detect microcalcifications due to their small sizes [14]. Yu and Guan [15] presented a method for the microcalcifications regions in mammography images. They first segmented the potential calcium-containing micro regions by means of mixed features and then extracted 31 features in order to obtain the real calcium-containing micro regions. The key feature of their method is the detection of microcalcifications. In another paper [16] authors presented an automatic tumor classification technique. They divided the initial images into several patches and extracted the features of these images by means of Gabor wavelets (using Gabor wavelets an image can be decomposed into several orientations. It is a frequently used texture analysis due to its discriminating features [17]). They subsequently used the principal component analysis to reduce the dimensions and employed support vector machine (SVM) as a classifier to grade the tumors. Although this method is able to separate the features related to the Gabor filter, this study just utilizes one classifier. Unlike the previous reference, a wide variety of classifiers were used for the classification of mammography images in [18], where the authors turned the problem of classifying mammography images into a one-class problem (normal class versus outliers) and exploited the Radon Generalized Transform to extract the image features (Radon transform is an integral transform which is used to reconstruct computerized tomography images. Its generalized form is defined on R^n Euclidean space [19]). In another attempt for dealing with diagnosis of breast cancer [20], several mammography images were segmented and then features were extracted based on the texture and boundaries of segmented regions. While the development of a feature selection method for mammography images is a major contribution of this study, it does not analyze the effects of different segmentation methods on the final accuracy. The authors of another study ([21]) used unbalanced data for training the hierarchy of features. They used an unsupervised sparse autoencoder with a new sparsity regularizer for training the extracted features. They successfully segmented breast density and also graded the breast tissue. Arevalo et al. [22] used a convolution neural networks (CNN) to train the features of mammography images and then employed the SVM method to classify the penultimate layer of CNN. Despite achieving high accuracy, it was better to use online datasets such as DDSM instead of dedicated datasets.

Applications of fuzzy techniques in image analysis are presented in [23]. The authors of [24] combined Gaussian mixture model with fuzzy logic. To benefit from fuzzy clustering methods, another article built on fuzzy c-means [25] to classify and estimate the level of breast compactness. They achieved 67.8% correct classification of fibroglandular and adipose. They divided mammography images into two groups of "fat" and "dense" to determine the parameter values for their methods, and used different values to each of these two groups. In another article [12], the authors used intuitionistic fuzzy sets (IFSs) to enhance mammography images. IFS generalizes fuzzy set theory, as its members are specified by using both the membership and non-membership definitions for the set. They first separated the breast tissue using the thresholding method and then fuzzified the image using intuitionistic fuzzy membership functions. Then they achieved a filtered image through manipulation of the background and foreground membership and defuzzification of the fuzzy plane. By fusing this image with the original image, the final upgraded image was obtained.

3   Algorithm Description

Figure 1 shows the output of our proposed algorithm at every step for a test image from the DDSM database. As it is observed, the presented algorithm includes 5 subsections, which will be subsequently explained.

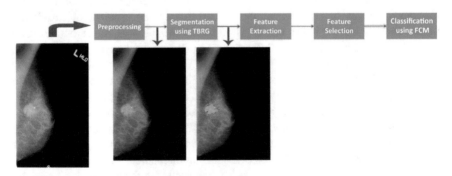

Fig. 1 Steps involved in the proposed algorithm

3.1 Preprocessing

Mammography images are inherently noisy because of the imaging process which uses high-energy radiation beams. The study in [26] regarding the amount of noise in mammography images attributes the source of noise in these images to the fluctuation of highly-energetic particles. Therefore, it is necessary to preprocess the acquired mammography images in order to reduce the effect of noise and other extraneous factors on the presented algorithm.

A three-step preprocessing has been employed here. In the first step, a median filter has been used to reduce the noise level. Median filters are widely used in noise removing due to their edge preservation property [27].

In the second step, the artifacts are eliminated from the images. Most of the mammography images contain patient names or MLO and CC labels. If these labels are close to the region of interest, they can adversely affect the segmentation and classification results. Consequently, we remove such artifacts by using a similar approach to [28]. Specifically, using the multilevel Otsu method, 16 threshold levels $t_1...t_{16}$ corresponding to classes $C_1...C_{16}$ are obtained for the images. The interclass variance for classes $C_1...C_{16}$ is obtained from Eq. 1.

$$\sigma_{BW}^2 = \sum_{t=1}^{16} P_t(m_t - m_G)^2 \tag{1}$$

In Eq. 1, σ_{BW}^2 is the interclass variance, P_t is the cumulative probability that a pixel is a member of the tth class, m_t is the mean brightness intensity of the tth class, and m_G (i.e. global mean) is the mean brightness intensity of the whole mammography image. According to the properties of the Otsu method, the thresholds of $t_1...t_{16}$ are chosen such that the class members will have the maximum interclass variance.

Next, by using the smallest member of $t_1...t_{16}$, the mammography image is binarized. Finally, by using an area opening morphological operator the regions with an area smaller than an arbitrary threshold area in the binarized image are eliminated. The area opening morphological operator consists of an erosion following a dilation. It is mainly supposed to eliminate micro spots of the image emerging as noise. A closing operator can also be used to fill in the holes. By multiplying this image by the original mammography image, the preprocessed image is obtained.

The third, and the last, preprocessing step involves the sub-sampling of images. Due to the large dimensions of the existing images in the DDSM database, the segmentation process could take a long time. For this reason, the images are sub-sampled by a factor of 4. Other cases were also analyzed for subsampling; however, they did not have significant results, something which was confirmed by [29], too. Thus, it can be an appropriate choice to reduce the algorithm learning time. Figure 1 shows an output of preprocessing step for a mammography image.

3.2   Segmentation

The segmentation step can greatly affect the ultimate precision of the algorithm; because a lack of proper segmentation may lead to the extraction of inadequate features based on the segmented regions and may undermine the efficacy of the whole process.

In this subsection we describe a new segmentation algorithm called the TBRG algorithm. The tumors showing up in mammography images are lighter in color than their surrounding tissue. Also, a severe difference between the brightness levels of two regions may indicate the presence of a tumor [30]. Thus, the average brightness level of a tumor is expected to be higher than that of the surrounding tissue, and also the variance of the brightness levels is expected to increase as we move away from the tumor. Therefore, if a balance could be created between average brightness and variance, a tumor can be segmented. This is exactly what the proposed TBRG algorithm does. This algorithm has 4 steps which are described in Algorithm 1.

Algorithm 1: TBGR segmentation method

1. Create a First In First Out (FIFO) memory F
2. Add to F a seed point determined by a radiologist/expert (typically the tumor's center)
3. Initialize the threshold $I_{th_{new}}$ to:
 	
$$I_{th_{new}} = \frac{1}{8}\sum_{i=1}^{8} I(p(i))$$
 	
    3.1. while F is not empty
               3.1.1. for every neighbor p* of pixel p in F
                     if I(p*) $> I_{th_{new}}$
                         add p* to segmented region
                         add neighbors of p* to F
               3.1.2. remove p from F
    3.2. set $I_{th_{old}} = I_{th_{new}}$
    3.3. set $I_{th_{new}} = I_{th_{old}} - \alpha \times Average + \beta \times Variance$
  While $I_{th_{new}} - I_{th_{old}} > \xi$
4. Using the area opening morphological operator to eliminate the noises arising from the
    segmentation process.
5. Save segmented region

In Algorithm 1, I(p(i)) is the intensity of ith neighbor of seed point. In the initialization phase of the F, seed point will be added to it. I(p^*) denotes the intensity of pixel p^*. Average and Variance notations which are used in the step 3.3 of Algorithm 1 show the average and variance of the intensities of the pixels which are located inside the segmented region.

During segmentation by the TBRG algorithm, points of very low brightness may exist within a tumor, which can lead to noise in the segmented region in the form of dark tiny points. Step 4 of the algorithm deals with such a problem.

The only point left regarding the TBRG algorithm is the adjustment of parameters α, β and ξ. For determining the values of these parameters, two different methods are suggested:

Experimental: In this approach a radiologist is needed as a specialist. The free parameters of the TBRG algorithm are adjusted manually and the segmentation outcome is shown to the radiologist. This procedure is repeated many times until the segmented images have minimum difference with ground truth.

Evolutionary-based algorithms: The values of free parameters α, β and ξ can be found by applying evolutionary algorithms (EAs) such as PSO or genetic algorithms. In this approach, we need an objective function in addition to the ground truth of images. The ground truth can be obtained through manual segmentation using the opinions of experts. Moreover, the DDSM dataset presents the ground truth of all the images as a default. The objective function for optimization can be defined as Eq. 2:

$$min \sum_{Z=1}^{T} \sum_{i=0}^{M} \sum_{j=0}^{N} (X_Z(i,j) - Y_Z(i \cdot j))^2 \qquad (2)$$

where T is the total number of images in the training set, M and N are the length and width of the Zth image in the database, respectively. $X_Z(i,j)$ is the brightness intensity of the segmented pixel of the Zth image at (i,j) coordinates and $Y_Z(i,j)$ is the intensity of the ground truth pixel of the Zth image at (i,j) coordinates.

Jacard index can also be used in addition to the existing function in Eq. 3. Jacard index, defined by Eq. 3, specifies the degree of similarity of two set. The value of Jacard index varies within the interval [0, 1] where 0 and 1 indicate the highest and lowest degrees of similarity, respectively.

$$J(A \cdot B) = \frac{|A \cap B|}{|A \cup B|} \qquad (3)$$

In the above equation, J(A,B) represents the Jacard index for two sets of A and B, $|A \cap B|$ denotes the number of members in set $A \cap B$, and $|A \cup B|$ indicates the number of members in set $A \cup B$. In the context of our work, A represents a ground truth image (i.e. manually segmented image by radiologists) and B shows a segmented image obtained by running TBRG algorithm. So $|A \cap B|$ denotes the number of pixels which are inside a tumor region in both A and B. In contrast, $|A \cup B|$ denotes the number of pixels which are inside a tumor region in both A and B plus the number of pixels which are in one image but not the other.

In this research, we have an employed evolutionary-based approach and used Eq. 3 as the objective function. Specifically, we used the PSO method. It should be noted that, when applying the PSO method to get the 3 unknown parameters of α, β

Table 1 Description of free parameters of Algorithms 1 and 2

Parameter	Description	Range
α	Weight of average in similarity measurement of Algorithm 1	[0.01, 0.05] in 8-bit images
β	Weight of variance in similarity measurement of Algorithm 1	[0.01, 0.05] in 8-bit images
ξ	Convergence threshold of Algorithm 1	[1, 3] in 8-bit images
K	Halting criterion threshold of Algorithm 2	[5, 15]

and ξ, we just used the training set. Functions and ranges of all free parameters of Algorithm 1 are outlined in Table 1.

Determining the correct range of parameters is very important, e.g. if α in Algorithm 1 is set lower than 0.01, it lead our proposed algorithm to output a single pixel.

We visualize the output of a segmentation step in Fig. 1 for the mammography image. A 66% Jacard index was obtained for this image.

3.3 Feature Extraction

We extracted 36 features describing boundary and texture of segment area. They are detailed in Appendix.

3.4 Feature Selection

The goal of feature selection is to select a subset of existing features, which has as few members as possible and which does not degrade the classification accuracy. There is a variety of feature selection methods, including the backward, forward or floating search feature selection.

The feature selection approach employed here is an improved version of [31], where our novelty is on using continuous PSO algorithm instead of the binary one. This method comprises two steps. In step 1, a 36×1 vector is considered as the optimization variables, with each of its members having a value between [0.2–0.4]. Equation 4 specifies whether a feature exists or not.

$$f(x_i) = \begin{cases} 0 & x_i < 0.3 \\ 1 & x_i \geq 0.3 \end{cases} \tag{4}$$

where, x_i denotes the ith feature, and 0 or 1 indicates the absence or the presence of the ith feature, respectively. In this step, continuous PSO algorithm has converged to a vector which contains 14 members with the values above 0.3. So in the first step of feature selection, in order to have minimum validation error, we have chosen these 14 features as the primary output of feature selection method.

However, number of obtained features is not necessarily minimum. The objective for step 2 is to consider the number of features as a part of the optimization process as well. For doing so, a 14×1 vector is chosen as the optimization variables, and the presence or absence of these variables in the final model is determined by Eq. 5. The optimization function in this step is defined as Eq. 5.

$$f = \gamma \times \frac{\#features}{\#AllFeatures} + (1 - \gamma) \times \frac{ErrorRate}{ER} \tag{5}$$

Here, γ is a constant factor in the interval [0, 1], '#features' indicates the number of selected features, '#AllFeatures' shows the total number of features, 'ErrorRate' denotes the error of training or validation resulted by using the selected features and 'ER' represents the training or validation error for the whole set of features. In the end, 8 features are selected.

3.5 Classification Using Fuzzy Cognitive Maps

FCMs model a causal system as a set of concepts and causal relationships between these concepts. As another chapter is dedicated to FCMs, we will briefly note that we use the following sigmoid transfer function (as in [32]):

$$f(x) = \frac{1}{1 + e^{-\eta x}} \tag{6}$$

where η is a parameter which determines steepness of f(x). Typical value of η is 5 [33].

3.5.1 FCM Classification Process

To construct our proposed model, the features selected in the previous step are considered as FCM concepts. That is, for each of the eight features chosen by the feature selection step, there is one corresponding FCM concept. We also added a concept as the output of the model. In total, we have nine concepts. After convergence of FCM, classification of an input sample is done by the means of a score which was obtained from output concept.

To increase the accuracy of the classification, a new method is proposed based on the PSO and the area under curve (AUC) value of the output concept. Algorithm 2 describes how we train our FCM.

---

1. Initialize FCM and PSO algorithm.

2. While fitness value is not constant in K iterations

       2.1. for every training sample
             2.1.1. enter the sample to the FCM
             2.1.2. for t=1 to 20
                      calculate $C_i(t)$ for all concepts by Eq. 6
             2.1.3. if $|C_i(t) - C_i(t-1)| < 0.001$ for all C_i
                      save the value of C_{out}
       2.2. if $|C_i(t+1) - C_i(t)| < 0.001$ for all C_i and for all training samples
                      calculate $\int_0^1 ROC(FPr)dFPr$ (AUC) of the saved values of C_{out}
                      set calculated AUC as the output of fitness function and return it to PSO
                      obtain new weights from PSO
         else if $|C_i(t+1) - C_i(t)| \not< 0.001$ for at least a C_i and for at least a training sample
                      let output of fitness function = -100
                      obtain new weights from PSO

3. Save the weights with maximum value of fitness.

Algorithm 2: Steps of FCM classification process

In the initialization phase of Algorithm 2, a fully connected and bidirectional FCM with an output concept is considered. To initialize the first population in the PSO algorithm, we generate several random weight matrices (as many as the population size set to 100) whose entries are in the range $[-1, 1]$. In step 2.2, if the values of concepts become oscillating (limit-cycles) or chaotic, a large negative value is returned to the PSO algorithm, instead of AUC of the output concept, to be able to move away from the subspace of non-optimal weights. Furthermore, the parameter k in second step of Algorithm 2 is a threshold which determines when the algorithm stops. Its typical value is shown in Table 1.

Figure 2 shows the general scheme of learning process used for classification with FCMs.

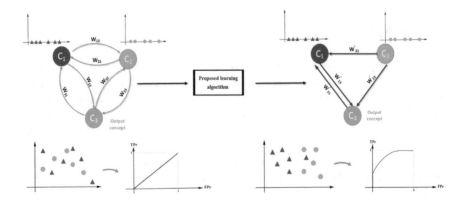

Fig. 2 Generic process of classification using the propose FCM learning algorithm

4 Experimental Results

The method described in Sect. 3, including preprocessing method, TBRG segmentation algorithm and proposed FCM learning algorithm, was implemented using Matlab v. 2016b.

To evaluate the efficacy of the proposed method, it was tested on the 'Benign01' and 'Cancer01' datasets of DDSM database [34], which contain mammography images for 139 female patients. The labels (MLO, CC) are included in the image for each patient. In addition, the existing tumors in the mammography images contained in this database have been manually segmented by radiologists.

We have performed 10-fold cross validation. The results of our FCM, with weights trained using our proposed PSO evolutionary algorithm, are shown in Fig. 3 and Table 2. We also designed two scenarios to compare our approach with other methods.

The aim of the first scenario was to compare the power of FCM directly with other conventional classifiers. Thus, the proposed method (Sect. 3) was employed for SVM, KNN, and LDA. Then the greedy search was used to optimize the free parameters of these classifiers separately. Table 3 reports the accuracy of aforementioned classifiers by applying 10-fold cross-validation to the entire data. Figure 3 indicates the ROC curves of FCM, SVM, KNN, and LDA together. According to Table 3 and Fig. 3, our FCM worked well as a classifier.

The aim of the second scenario was to compare the proposed approach with other methods in accuracy. In this scenario, certain references were selected due to the use of a similar database and their results are depicted in Table 4.

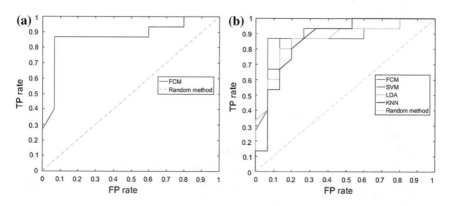

Fig. 3 ROC curves **a** FCM which is trained using Algorithm 1, and **b** other classifiers

Table 2 Results of classification for FCM which is trained using Algorithm 2

	Accuracy	Sensitivity	Specificity	MCC	AUC
	88.33%	86.66%	90%	0.7670	87.11%

Table 3 Results of classification for SVM, LDA and KNN

	Accuracy (%)	Sensitivity (%)	Specificity (%)	MCC (%)	AUC (%)
LDA	83.33	80	86.66	0.6681	86.22
SVM	86.66	86.66	86.66	0.7333	86.44
KNN	80	80	80	0.60	86.00

Table 4 Classification performance of different methods on DDSM database

Reference	Method	Sensitivity	Specificity	Accuracy	AUC
This work	FCM	86.66%	90%	88.33%	0.87
Li et al. [35]	Texton analysis	85.48%	86.54%	85.96%	0.92
Chokri and Farida [10]	Multi-layer perceptron with manually segmented images	82.76%	90.3%	88.02%	–
Surendiran and Vadivel [36]	Step wise analysis of variance discriminant analysis	84.7%	90%	87%	–
Choi et al. [37]	Ensemble learning with neural network as base classifier	–	–	–	0.86
Choi et al. [37]	Ensemble learning with SVM as base classifier	–	–	–	0.87
Jiao et al. [38]	Deep convolutional neural networks	–	–	92.5%	–

According to Table 4, our proposed approach produced better results than [10, 35] and [36] with respect to accuracy. Given the number of free parameters used by CNN in [38], that classifier showed a higher level of accuracy than our proposed approach. However, it should be noted that increasing the number of parameters increases the probability of overfitting. Regarding sensitivity, our method produced better results than other methods mentioned in Table 4.

5 Conclusion

Because of the high mortality of breast cancer patients, it is necessary to develop algorithms that can help in the early detection of breast tumors. In this regard, an algorithm was presented in this chapter for detecting and classifying breast tumors into benign and cancerous types. This algorithm consists of 5 steps: preprocessing, segmentation by means of a new TBRG algorithm, feature extraction, feature selection and FCM-based classification.

The TBRG algorithm is a new member of a region growing family of algorithms and it attempts to segment mammography images by striking a balance between the mean and variance of brightness intensity within a tumor region. The empirical results obtained by applying the presented algorithm in this chapter indicate the achievement of 87.11% AUC in the test set by the TBRG algorithm in combination with FCM. Through comparisons of our proposed method with typical classifiers, as well as other methods tested on the same dataset, we concluded that our method has high accuracy and potential for future developments. In future works, with regards to the features of an input image, the free parameters of TBRG algorithm could be investigated by adapting their values in order to increase the calculated Jacard index.

Appendix

In this appendix, the features extracted from the segmented images are described. A total of 36 features that describe the texture and the boundaries of the segmented region were extracted. The designations of these features are given in Table 5, followed by a brief explanation regarding each extracted feature.

1. Circularity

The circularity of a region, which shows its resemblance to a circle, is obtained from Eq. (7)

$$Circularity = \frac{P^2}{A} \tag{7}$$

Here, P and A denote the circumference and the area of a segmented region, respectively.

2. Area

The area of a segmented region is equal to the total number of pixels which are members of this region.

Table 5 Names of the extracted features

1	Circularity	7	Second invariant moment
2	Area	8	Entropy of contour gradient
3	Features related to radial length (2 features)	9	Average brightness intensity
4	Entropy	10	Standard deviation of brightness intensity
5	Features related to fractal index (3 features)	11	Features related to GLCM (14 features)
6	Eccentricity	12	Simplified version of histogram of gradient (9 features)

3. Features related to radial length

In order to determine this feature, it is necessary to first obtain the center of the segmented region by Eq. (8). Then the Euclidean distance of each pixel on the contour (Boundary of the segmented region) is calculated from the geometrical center. The average and the standard deviation of these distances constitute the two features of this section.

$$X = \frac{1}{N} \sum_{i=1}^{N} x_i. \quad Y = \frac{1}{N} \sum_{i=1}^{N} y_i \tag{8}$$

Here, N is the number of pixels on the contour, x_i and y_i are the x,y coordinates of the ith pixel on the contour, and X and Y are the x, y coordinates of the segmented region's geometrical center.

4. Entropy of the segmented region

The entropy of the segmented region's brightness intensity is obtained from Eq. (9). The entropy is a measure of the randomness of a random variable.

$$E = - \sum_{i=1}^{N} p_i \log(p_i) \tag{9}$$

where, N denotes the number of brightness levels and p_i is the probability of having a pixel with brightness level i in the segmented region.

5. Features related to fractal index

By measuring the variations of details with respect to scale, fractal dimension can provide a criterion for the complexity of a segmented region [39]. The fractal dimension of a segmented region can be computed by means of Eq. (10).

$$N = N_0 R^{-D} \tag{10}$$

Here, N denotes the number of boxes superimposed to the segmented area, N_0 is an arbitrary constant, R is the size of different boxes and D is the fractal dimension. N and R can be obtained by using the box counting method [40]. In view of Eq. (10), if the $\log^N$-$\log^R$ diagram is modeled on a line, the slope (i.e. the fractal dimension) and the intercept of this line can be used as two features. Also, the dispersion variance of the slopes of lines in the $\log^N$-$\log^R$ diagram could be considered as another feature.

6. Eccentricity

Eccentricity shows the degree of lengthening of the segmented region [41], and it is obtained from the eigenvalues of Matrix A whose entries can be defined with regards to Eq. (11).

$$A_{11} = \sum_{i=1}^{N} (x_i - X)^2 \cdot A_{22} = \sum_{i=1}^{N} (y_i - Y)^2 \cdot A_{12} = A_{21} = \sum_{i=1}^{N} (x_i - X)(y_i - Y) \qquad (11)$$

In the above equation, A_{ij} is the entry related to the ith row and jth column of Matrix A, N is the number of pixels on the boundary, x_i and y_i represent the coordinates of the ith pixel on the boundary, and X and Y denote the coordinates of the segmented region's geometrical center.

7. Second invariant moment

The second and the third moments of an image can be defined so that they are robust against variables like rotation and scale. A number of these moments have been introduced in [42]. We have extracted the second invariant moment as a feature for the segmented region.

8. Entropy of contour gradient

For extracting this feature, by using the Sobel operator, the gradient direction of the pixels on the segmented region's boundary is determined. Then, by considering this gradient direction and Fig. 4, the histogram of gradient direction is obtained for the 8-neighbor case, and by 8 bins.

After establishing the gradient direction histogram, the entropy of contour gradient can be obtained from Eq. (12).

$$E = - \sum_{i=1}^{8} p_i \log(p_i) \qquad (12)$$

where, p_i is the probability of finding an arbitrary pixel on the boundary with maximum fluctuations in the direction of histogram's ith bin.

9. Average brightness intensity

The mean brightness intensity of the segmented region is extracted as a feature.

Fig. 4 The bins of gradient direction histogram for the case of 8 neighbors (each bin covers a total of 45°)

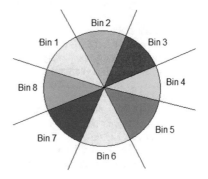

10. Standard deviation of brightness intensity

The standard deviation of the brightness intensities of the pixels within the segmented region is extracted as a feature.

11. Features related to GLCM

The grey level co-occurrence matrix (GLCM) has been extensively used to describe the image textures. In order to extract the features associated with GLCM, the tumor tissue texture is extracted by using the bounding box method, and then the GLCM matrix is determined for this region. Subsequently, 14 features are extracted, which are definable from this matrix.

12. Histogram of gradients

In this approach, which is the simplified method of the histogram of oriented gradients [43], the whole texture of the segmented region is extracted first by using the bounding box method, and the extracted image is considered as a cell. For this cell, a 9-bin histogram is obtained by considering the size and gradient direction of the existing pixels and these bins are used as features.

References

1. U.S. Breast cancer statistics (2017). http://www.breastcancer.org/symptoms/understand_bc/statistics
2. Ohuchi N, Suzuki A, Sobue T et al (2016) Sensitivity and specificity of mammography and adjunctive ultrasonography to screen for breast cancer in the Japan strategic anti-cancer randomized trial (J-START): a randomised controlled trial. Lancet 387:341–348
3. Kemp Jacobsen K, O'meara ES, Key D, et al (2015) Comparing sensitivity and specificity of screening mammography in the United States and Denmark. Int J Cancer 137:2198–2207
4. Du K-L, Swamy MNS (2016) Particle swarm optimization. In: Search and optimization by metaheuristics. Springer, pp 153–173
5. Mandal D, Chatterjee A, Maitra M (2017) Particle swarm optimization based fast Chan-Vese algorithm for medical image segmentation. In: Metaheuristics for medicine and biology. Springer, pp 49–74
6. Mustra M, Grgic M, Rangayyan RM (2016) Review of recent advances in segmentation of the breast boundary and the pectoral muscle in mammograms. Med Biol Eng Comput 54:1003–1024
7. de Oliveira Silva LC, Barros AK, Lopes MV (2017) Detecting masses in dense breast using independent component analysis. Artif Intell Med 80:29–38
8. Amirkhani A, Papageorgiou EI, Mohseni A, Mosavi MR (2017) A review of fuzzy cognitive maps in medicine: taxonomy, methods, and applications. Comput Methods Programs Biomed 142:129–145
9. Strand F, Humphreys K, Cheddad A et al (2016) Novel mammographic image features differentiate between interval and screen-detected breast cancer: a case-case study. Breast Cancer Res 18:100
10. Chokri F, Farida MH (2016) Mammographic mass classification according to Bi-RADS lexicon. IET Comput Vis 11:189–198

11. Rouhi R, Jafari M, Kasaei S, Keshavarzian P (2015) Benign and malignant breast tumors classification based on region growing and CNN segmentation. Expert Syst Appl 42:990–1002

12. Deng H, Deng W, Sun X et al (2017) Mammogram enhancement using intuitionistic fuzzy sets. IEEE Trans Biomed Eng 64:1803–1814

13. Jenifer S, Parasuraman S, Kadirvelu A (2016) Contrast enhancement and brightness preserving of digital mammograms using fuzzy clipped contrast-limited adaptive histogram equalization algorithm. Appl Soft Comput 42:167–177

14. Vivona L, Cascio D, Fauci F, Raso G (2014) Fuzzy technique for microcalcifications clustering in digital mammograms. BMC Med Imaging 14:23. https://doi.org/10.1186/1471-2342-14-23

15. Yu S, Guan L (2000) A CAD system for the automatic detection of clustered microcalcifications in digitized mammogram films. IEEE Trans Med Imaging 19:115–126

16. Buciu I, Gacsadi A (2011) Directional features for automatic tumor classification of mammogram images. Biomed Signal Process Control 6:370–378

17. Arivazhagan S, Ganesan L, Priyal SP (2006) Texture classification using Gabor wavelets based rotation invariant features. Pattern Recognit Lett 27:1976–1982

18. Ganesan K, Acharya UR, Chua CK et al (2014) One-class classification of mammograms using trace transform functionals. IEEE Trans Instrum Meas 63:304–311

19. Deans SR (2007) The Radon transform and some of its applications. Courier Corporation

20. Liu X, Tang J (2014) Mass classification in mammograms using selected geometry and texture features, and a new SVM-based feature selection method. IEEE Syst J 8:910–920

21. Kallenberg M, Petersen K, Nielsen M et al (2016) Unsupervised deep learning applied to breast density segmentation and mammographic risk scoring. IEEE Trans Med Imaging 35:1322–1331

22. Arevalo J, González FA, Ramos-Pollán R et al (2016) Representation learning for mammography mass lesion classification with convolutional neural networks. Comput Methods Programs Biomed 127:248–257

23. Kerre EE, Nachtegael M (2013) Fuzzy techniques in image processing. Physica

24. Aminikhanghahi S, Shin S, Wang W et al (2017) A new fuzzy Gaussian mixture model (FGMM) based algorithm for mammography tumor image classification. Multimed Tools Appl 76:10191–10205

25. Pavan ALM, Vacavant A, Trindade AP, de Pina DR (2017) Fibroglandular tissue quantification in mammography by optimized fuzzy C-means with variable compactness. IRBM 38:228–233

26. Goebel PM, Belbachir AN, Truppe M (2005) Noise estimation in panoramic X-ray images: An application analysis approach. In: 2005 IEEE/SP 13th workshop on statistical signal processing, pp 996–1001

27. Hsieh M-H, Cheng F-C, Shie M-C, Ruan S-J (2013) Fast and efficient median filter for removing 1–99% levels of salt-and-pepper noise in images. Eng Appl Artif Intell 26:1333–1338

28. Qayyum A, Basit A (2016) Automatic breast segmentation and cancer detection via SVM in mammograms. In: 2016 International conference on emerging technologies (ICET), pp 1–6

29. Tourassi GD, Vargas-Voracek R, Catarious DM, Floyd CE (2003) Computer-assisted detection of mammographic masses: a template matching scheme based on mutual information. Med Phys 30:2123–2130

30. Lau T-K, Bischof WF (1991) Automated detection of breast tumors using the asymmetry approach. Comput Biomed Res 24:273–295

31. Xue B, Zhang M, Browne WN (2012) New fitness functions in binary particle swarm optimisation for feature selection. In: 2012 IEEE congress on evolutionary computation (CEC), pp 1–8

32. Bueno S, Salmeron JL (2009) Benchmarking main activation functions in fuzzy cognitive maps. Expert Syst Appl 36:5221–5229

33. Grant D, Osei-Bryson K-M (2005) Using fuzzy cognitive maps to assess MIS organizational change impact. In: Proceedings of the 38th annual Hawaii international conference on system sciences, HICSS'05, 2005, p 263c–263c
34. Heath M, Bowyer K, Kopans D et al (2000) The digital database for screening mammography. In: Proceedings of the 5th international workshop on digital mammography. pp 212–218
35. Li Y, Chen H, Rohde GK et al (2015) Texton analysis for mass classification in mammograms. Pattern Recognit Lett 52:87–93
36. Surendiran B, Vadivel A (2010) Feature selection using stepwise ANOVA discriminant analysis for mammogram mass classification. Int J Recent Trends Eng Technol 3:55–57
37. Choi JY, Kim DH, Plataniotis KN, Ro YM (2016) Classifier ensemble generation and selection with multiple feature representations for classification applications in computer-aided detection and diagnosis on mammography. Expert Syst Appl 46:106–121
38. Jiao Z, Gao X, Wang Y, Li J (2016) A deep feature based framework for breast masses classification. Neurocomputing 197:221–231
39. Mandelbrot B (1982) The fractal geometry of nature. WH Freeman
40. Foroutan-pour K, Dutilleul P, Smith DL (1999) Advances in the implementation of the box-counting method of fractal dimension estimation. Appl Math Comput 105:195–210
41. Cascio D, Fauci F, Magro R et al (2006) Mammogram segmentation by contour searching and mass lesions classification with neural network. IEEE Trans Nucl Sci 53:2827–2833
42. Gonzalez RC, Woods RE (2002) Digital image processing. Prentice hall
43. Dalal N, Triggs B (2005) Histograms of oriented gradients for human detection. In: IEEE computer society conference on computer vision and pattern recognition, CVPR 2005. pp 886–893

Text-Based Analytics for Biosurveillance

Lauren E. Charles, William Smith, Jeremiah Rounds
and Joshua Mendoza

Abstract The ability to prevent, mitigate, or control a biological threat depends on how quickly the threat is identified and characterized. Ensuring the timely delivery of data and analytics is an essential aspect of providing adequate situational awareness in the face of a disease outbreak. This chapter outlines an analytic pipeline for supporting an advanced early warning system that can integrate multiple data sources and provide situational awareness of potential and occurring disease situations. The pipeline includes real-time automated data analysis founded on natural language processing, semantic concept matching, and machine learning techniques, to enrich content with metadata related to biosurveillance. Online news articles are presented as a use case for the pipeline, but the processes can be generalized to any textual data. In this chapter, the mechanics of a streaming pipeline are briefly discussed as well as the major steps required to provide targeted situational awareness. The text-based analytic pipeline includes various processing steps as well as identifying article relevance to biosurveillance (e.g., relevance algorithm) and article feature extraction (who, what, where, why, how, and when).

L. E. Charles (✉) · W. Smith · J. Rounds · J. Mendoza
Pacific Northwest National Laboratory, Richland, WA 99354, USA
e-mail: lauren.charles@pnnl.gov

W. Smith
e-mail: william.smith@pnnl.gov

J. Rounds
e-mail: jeremiah.rounds@pnnl.gov

J. Mendoza
e-mail: joshua.mendoza@pnnl.gov

© Springer International Publishing AG, part of Springer Nature 2018   117
P. J. Giabbanelli et al. (eds.), *Advanced Data Analytics in Health*, Smart Innovation,
Systems and Technologies 93, https://doi.org/10.1007/978-3-319-77911-9_7

1 Software Engineering and Architecture

This chapter is focused on the types of analytics that drive use of textual data for biosurveillance and touches upon the technologies that bridge together these analytics. Here is an overview of the suggested principles and technologies that can be used to create a successful biosurveillance system to support advanced early warning, integrate multiple data sources, and provide situational awareness of potential and occurring disease situations.

The overarching principles of the software system should focus on robustness yet flexibility in accommodating future needs and minimization of technologies, i.e., the best available to address the widest set of required features. We focus on stream processing pipelines that follow a Flow-Based Programming (FBP) paradigm [1]. In a valid data flow graph pipeline architecture, data flows from node 1 to node 2, where a node represents a pipeline process without any additional incoming or outgoing data [2]. To allow for easier integration, Eichenlberger et al. [2] created a user interface tool to visualize the pipeline, which allows the users to easily piece nodes (processes) together. There are several open source libraries for distributed computing packages to build such pipelines, including three Apache tools: NiFi to direct the flow of data, Storm to process the data, and Kafka for storing the data [3]. The reason for choosing an FBP paradigm is because the data pipeline (i.e., data ingestion, processing, and storage) supports a dynamic, disparate environment and lays the groundwork for cutting-edge efforts moving forward. This method decreases the cost and complexities of data integration yet increases the capacity for early warning, situational awareness, and operational relevance.

In practice, the Apache NiFi framework has proven very successful in the health surveillance setting. The NiFi framework supports consuming, processing, and distributing data to and from many diverse mechanisms through the concept of processors. For example, NiFi can access pull data available via HTTP (e.g., RSS feed) or consume a message queue system (e.g., Apache Kafka). NiFi can support push models, such as archived data (e.g., zip file pushed to a server) or a file watch system that detects when a new file is added for processing. If the required method to access data is not already developed, the framework is extensible and custom processors can easily be created to support the processing of most data sources or data formats. NiFi meets the eight requirements of a real-time stream process pipeline, which helps ensure that a system can handle a variety of real-time processing applications [4]. This allows NiFi to be used as an efficient Extract Transform and Load (ETL) pipeline that follows the FBP paradigm. Using NiFi, we can accomplish a variety of tasks ranging from basic routing of documents by properties to using complex backend databases, such as Elasticsearch for storing, searching, and aggregating data. These features, including NiFi's modular processors, allow for efficient pipeline updates and delivery of cutting-edge results.

In a real-time data pipeline, the data is continuously flowing from ingestion, processing to storage without system bottlenecks preventing ingestion of new data.

Examples of streaming analytic steps are formatting date and time, detecting language, entity extraction, natural language processing (NLP), converting formats, and adding metadata. For this phase of the pipeline, several technological options are available, e.g., AWS Lambda, Apache NiFi, Apache Storm, Apache Flink, or Spark. Apache NiFi is again a great candidate for processes that are fast and work on a single unit of data at a time. The technology scales linearly and horizontally, meaning as additional computing resources are added, there is a one-to-one improvement in performance and computing resources can be spread across many machines in the form of a cluster. For state-full processing analytics, i.e., a single unit of data is part of a larger data process, a distributed compute platform, such as Apache Storm, should be used. Examples of a state-full process are maintaining a sliding window of counts over the last hour and determining a data trend based on what has already come in. Through this mechanism, real-time alerting can be supported.

2 Text-Based Analytic Pipeline

The following analytic pipeline outlines a use case of characterizing web-based articles for biosurveillance purposes. A NiFi framework has been used to process documents through the various analytic steps (Fig. 1).

2.1 Article Relevance

The goal of this step is to identify web-based articles that are relevant to biosurveillance to enable real-time situational awareness of global health. Here, articles are harvested as potential candidates through various sources, such as RSS feeds, specific source URLS, and Google alerts. The NiFi pipeline processes incoming articles into Javascript Object Notation (JSON) format and each data packet contains the initial article data and associated metadata, i.e., the title, short summary or gist, date, and source URL. JSON format is ideal in this setting; it is a human-readable, easily manipulated, and light-weight data-interchange format.

Natural Language Processing I. As an article enters the pipeline, the text must be quantified before analyses. The process of converting a text into usable data for analyses is called natural language processing (NLP). The most common way to quantify the article is by representing the text in a vector space. First, the articles' title and gist are broken into individual words, i.e., *tokens*. Various methods are available for converting document tokens into vectors, including using individual words, e.g., bag-of-words (BoW), term-frequency-inverse document frequency, or chunk parsers, e.g., n-grams of words. For the most flexibility in data manipulation, BoW vectors are used to represent the articles' title and gist fields. The text is

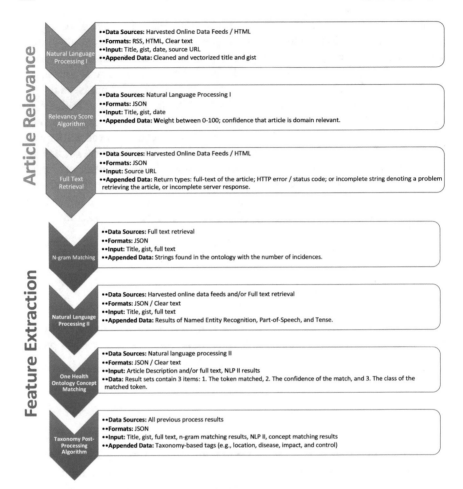

Fig. 1 Biosurveillance Health Analytics Pipeline Overview. The contextual flow of steps from harvesting web-based articles to article presentation to an analyst for surveillance purposes. Data sources, formats, input, and the appended data from each step are described

simplified to a set of words (i.e., bag) that retains word multiplicity but ignores grammar and word order. This method enables the frequency of word occurrence to be used as a feature in training document classifiers. Here, the title and gist contribute to distinct BoW feature vector for each document. Keeping these counts separated allows algorithms to place a different importance on the two document elements.

In effort to reduce the resulting vector space, the data vector undergoes stop word removal and word stemming procedures. By filtering out *stop words*, words that are irrelevant or do not provide any more contextual meaning to the vector space are removed. For example, words, such as "a", "the", "this" or "is", are extremely common in natural language but are not relevant to concept matching or mapping. *Stem* refers to the part of the word left over when the affix and suffix are removed. Stemming algorithms identify the stem of a collective group of words that have similar meanings, e.g., infected, infection, and infectious all stem to the word infect, to boost the frequency of concepts identified.

Further processing of BoW can be done as feature engineering [5]. In the pipeline described, this step is left to algorithms that utilize the BoW feature sets. Features can be extracted that are not just word counts. For example, paragraph organization and sentence length can play a role in scoring a documents relevancy [6]. In addition, BoW is a unigram procedure that can be extended to bi-grams and n-grams feature vectors. Dimension reduction techniques can be applied to BoW, e.g., word2vec [7]. The resulting processed list of tokens and data vector is saved in the article JSON packet for subsequent analysis.

2.1.1 Relevance Score Algorithm

The goal of this section is to identify the articles most relevant to biosurveillance and to filter out articles that were incidentally harvested. Training a machine learning algorithm to differentiate between relevant and irrelevant articles using only the title and gist of the articles keeps the analytic pipeline clean, decreasing computing time and congestion. There are many document classification algorithms (see Aggarwal and Zhai 2012 for a review) [8]. In this case, a penalized Logistic Regression model (PLR) is used due to the interpretability of output and portability of fit models. The PLR uses a BoW derived from concatenation of an article's title and gist [9]. The features are presence/absence of words re-weighted by inverse document frequency [10]. The algorithm, developed by modifying a spam filter [11] to specialized biosurveillance needs, scores documents as likely belonging either the irrelevant or relevant class, where relevant is defined as being important to a future/unknown user-interaction. The PLR output is a continuous log-odds that is used to calculate a relevancy score. As standard practice, the penalty in PLR is chosen with a 10-fold cross-validation procedure in training.

Training. The training set of documents are labeled as relevant or irrelevant. The relevant documents are articles deemed important by subject matter experts (SMEs). The irrelevant articles are identified through key terms, ex. "stock market" or "for sale", as well as by SMEs. Through topical analysis and clustering techniques on the harvested data, such as Latent Dirichlet Allocation, additional irrelevant key terms were identified and included in the irrelevant training dataset [12]. The training process must be updated regularly, e.g., monthly, to help identify new topics in the news that (1) may result in additional irrelevant articles being harvested by accident, e.g., a person's name or new clothing line, and (2) identify new relevant article language or disease topics of interest, e.g., new medicinal cure or disease name. This process can be performed either offline with subsequent uploading of the new model or directly with new labeled training documents incorporated into the pipeline; both processes are supported by the NiFi framework.

Retraining must include documents new to the current model to ensure timely, new topic identification.

Empirical Calibration and Scoring. Once the PLR model is trained and incorporated into the NiFi processor, the model appends a log-odds score (LOD) to the article metadata that indicates how relevant (high score) or irrelevant (low score) an article is to biosurveillance. Unfortunately, the value of continuous score responds to the prior proportion of classes in labeled training documents, which may not reflect the proportions for these documents in the entire feed. From a random sample of 100 k documents from the incoming feed, a mean, standard deviation, and empirical cumulative distribution function (CDF) for LODs are calculated. The LOD score is augmented with standardized LOD of relevancy (i.e., mean 0 and standard deviation of 1) and percentile LOD (i.e., the probability that a randomly sampled document LOD is less than or equal to the current document). These values are stored with the model for further processing.

Filtering and Ranking. Extreme cases of high and low values can be used to filter articles by importance. Those that are deemed with low scores are filtered out into a separate irrelevant database for use in the retraining set and quality assurance purposes to ensure relevant articles are not filtered out. The remaining articles and relevance score are passed through the pipeline to the next step. This relevancy score allows documents to be prioritized both for processing and for user consideration. For example, the relevancy score with time can parsimoniously rank documents that are both recent and relevant, e.g., Reddit.com hot-score [13]. For document relevancy, a relevancy-time score is calculated as the standardized LOD—(publication age in days)/(7 Days). When LOD values are greater than the 99th percentile, a threshold procedure is applied so that high-scoring outliers are replaced in rank by newer documents in a timely fashion.

2.1.2 Full Text Retrieval

The depth of information derived from an article depends on the length of the text available for mining. The title and gist of an article provide a highlight summary but the full article may contain vital information to situational awareness of the event. The text retrieval processor, i.e. web scraper, is designed to fetch online articles, remove the HTML markup, and conduct initial text cleaning before saving it as part of the associated article JSON object.

Online articles can be difficult to retrieve and parse because there are several conflicting techniques across websites for HTML markup and delivery. The content and layout of webpages is unpredictable, making text extraction from articles error-prone. In addition, there are some webpages that actively try to block downloading of text or change the content regularly via server calls invisible to a web scraper. Given the potential problems, the best approach includes minimal time between notification and retrieval of documents, identification of key websites of interest, and using a succession of methods to increase web coverage.

Reliable python packages, such as Newspaper and Goose, can provide a good amount of web coverage. However, for some webpages, a unique work around solution is required. For example, HTML content may appear "hidden" on webpages with a dynamically loaded Document Object Model structure. For these pages, a JavaScript request is required for the content to load and then be extracted. In other instances, websites require a fee to access their content. An alternative approach is a pay service to retrieve text, e.g., webscraper.io or Import.io.

2.2 Feature Extraction

Once the article has gone through initial processing steps, the next goal is to understand the content of an article and what role it plays in biosurveillance. This part of the pipeline appends the article JSON with a standardized list of information that can be used to summarize the article's relevance to biosurveillance.

To facilitate NLP analysis, the full text of the document is vectorized using the BoW method at the paragraph-level (see Sect. 2.1). By splitting up the articles by paragraph, coherent ideas are grouped together, which may get lost when mixed in with the whole document. The feature extraction techniques below (n-gram matching, NLP, and concept matching) are combined in a post-processing algorithm to create a conceptual outline of each article. The concepts extracted are standardized and based on the tagging schema below, developed specifically for a biosurveillance use-case, but can be fine-tuned for other applications.

2.2.1 Tagging Schema

There are several ways to identify concepts in text data. These range from clustering articles to identify topics based on similar words present in documents to a priori knowledge of topics of interest and then identifying articles containing those words or concepts. Both approaches are used in the analytic tasks, however, for different purposes. Clustering techniques are used for data mining of articles to identify types of topics that provide additional insight into the dataset [12]. For the analytic pipeline, a set of standard features to-be identified in the articles are represented in a tagging schema and techniques are applied to identify those concepts. The main tags categories are domain, subjects, location, grammatical tense, and specific biosurveillance topics.

The most general concepts to be extracted are the location and grammatical tense. There are standardized datasets that outline this type of information and are utilized in the pipeline. Location defines where an event has occurred, plays an important role in the epidemiology, and defines a biosurveillance analysts' areas of responsibility. Therefore, having a precise understanding of the locations mentioned in an article has a large impact on what the article is about. The location tagging schema comes from a gazetteer, which is a type of geographical dictionary that contains a hierarchical-like description of the names of places (e.g., obofoundry. org). The grammatical tense plays an important role in understanding the context of the article. The tense can be used to understand whether the article is describing a historical event (Past), something that is occurring now (Present), or describing a plan, such as implementing a new policy (Future).

General information associated with biosurveillance is present in the domain and subject tags. The domain tags simply describe the article's relationship to biology in the broadest sense, e.g., humans, animals, and pathogen type. The subject tags, on the other hand, are intended to include all potential broad-level subjects found in online bio-related documents. Therefore, a subject tagging schema was developed. Through a combination of SME knowledge and article cluster analysis, 3 overarching subjects with subcategories emerged: (1) Government-like topics related to (a) elections, (b) policy or (c) education; (2) Research-related to (a) theoretical, (b) medical products/treatment, or (c) conference/meeting; and (3) Event-related to (a) new, (b) ongoing, or (c) aftermath.

For topics focused on defining a disease event, an interdisciplinary SME-developed biosurveillance-related tagging schema was created. This schema represents a hierarchy of disease-related information used in biosurveillance and contains hundreds of standardized tags aimed at identifying key topics in an article. The main categories present in this topic tagging schema are etiologic agent, control measures, and public health impact.

By combing the separate tagging schemas described in this section, a standardized form of where, when, who, what, why, and how is systematically identified for each article. Subsequently, this information can be used to provide situational awareness, prediction, and, ultimately, prevention of disease outbreaks.

2.2.2 N-Gram Matching

N-Gram matching is a category of feature extraction techniques that ignores context and focuses on the literal comparisons of a set of search terms and those terms present in a document. Due to the simplicity of the method, the tagging schema is restricted to term-based tags (e.g., the location and biosurveillance-specific topic tags) rather than concept based tags (e.g., tense or subject). To increase method robustness, sets of synonyms for tag terms are collected, i.e., WordNet synsets, and linked to the same tag ID. These synsets are identified manually, through a lexical database, ontology, or software tools, such as WordNet [14]. The total number of tag IDs with their associated total counts per article are appended to the JSON. This metadata is used later in the taxonomy post-processing algorithm (see Sect. 2.2.5).

The most straightforward n-gram technique uses a BoW approach and performs a recursive n-gram matching algorithm. The process to matching is as follows: The maximum number of consecutive tokens, i.e., n-grams, required to parse the given text is equal to the largest number of tokens in a single search term within the set of search terms. Starting with the longest term in the set of search terms, a defined regular expression (generally case insensitive) attempts explicit matching on sentence tokens in the target text.

With user-defined n-gram tokens, the 1-to-1 concept matching can be removed from the programming environment and queried against a data store. This technique has two major differences from the regex programmatic comparison: 1. Query Language: By removing the match pattern from the programming environment, the system relies on a query language that the data store manufacture implements, generally only rudimentary regular expression transformations within the query. 2. Data Store/Set Optimization: Databases have an array of internal storage methods (e.g., Graph, Semantic RDF Graphs, Key-Value Pair, and ApacheLucene). The speed and breadth of recall is dependent on the manufacturer and implementation of internal storage algorithms.

ElasticSearch is a key-value store specifically built upon ApacheLucene for quick retrieval and matching. Here, 50 K available search tokens are stored within ElasticSearch and can be queried by class within each document n-gram for fast retrieval of 1-to-1 matches within the documents. Using ElasticSearch provides several matching algorithms depending on configuration), but these can be replicated programmatically or with different data store solutions. MongoDB is an example of a competing data store with similar query capabilities to ElasticSearch, but was not natively designed to match sets of tokens with full text queries. To compensate for this, MongoDB applications focus on the speed of retrieval while programmatically comparing the results instead of putting the full operation of query result comparison on the data store.

2.2.3 Natural Language Processing II

Further NLP efforts are required to better understand aspects of articles outside of their direct content or topics. For instance, n-gram matching may identify Zika virus as the primary topic of an article, but miss the location or other details because they are not written as expected. For example, the location may be a famous building, e.g., Eiffel Tower, with implied geographic coordinates of Paris, France and, therefore, not picked up by the gazetteer n-gram matching. Additional NLP functionality can help reveal these types of nuanced details in an article, which is needed for more concept-based tags, such as tense and location.

Named-entity Recognition (NER). Linguistic markers (e.g., location names, organizations, quantities, dates) usually require more than just directly processing of a document. This type of information extraction is known as NER. NER is often achieved by applying statistical methods in machine learning to train a model to identify how these topics are presented in the corpus of documents, i.e., biosurveillance-related articles. The following general process for NER development can be adapted to various domains of interest: (1) collect relevant terms to search for, (2) collect documents with free-text that contain these terms, (3) build a training set with labels for the relevant terms, and (4) train a NER (e.g., conditional random fields model) with (3) and save for future use.

For these types of models to succeed, a significant amount of labeled training data is needed. Fortunately, NER libraries are freely available online and provide datasets that cover a wide range of use cases. The most widely used and well-studied NER library was developed through the Standford University NLP group [15]. However, there are other alternatives that can be investigated, such as the MITIE toolkit (github.com/mit-nlp/MITIE). This toolkit can be used as a command-line tool like the Stanford NLP tool and has the benefit of being directly accessible through the Python programming language's natural language toolkit (NLTK) [16]. This Python compatibility provides flexibility in training and utilizing of the NER model as well as other NLP tasks. Additionally, there are other toolkits that have been developed using recurrent neural networks (RNN) as the tagging model instead of the popular conditional random fields (github.com/glample/tagger). RNN's have shown excellent results on many NLP tasks and may boost performance for many application areas [17]. However, these models come with the additional cost of requiring much more data for training than is often available for biomedical NER models.

Part-of-speech (POS) Tagging. Grammatical tense detection is a difficult problem in NLP but dovetails other well-studied areas, e.g., POS tagging. POS taggers assign the parts of speech, e.g., noun, verb, or adjective, to each word through various methods, e.g., Stanford Log-linear POS Tagger [18]. By utilizing POS taggers on processed documents, decision rules for determining the overall tense of an article can be implemented. These tenses need only to be coarse-grained, i.e., "past", "present", and "future", to provide insight into whether events described in an article are a historical recollection, a current issue, or predicted to occur.

Document Structure. By leveraging structural elements of a document, e.g., title, gist, or heading, better decisions can be made about event details or tags, e.g., tense and location. For example, the header of an article may contain more relevant information about an event than a paragraph near the end of the article. By leveraging the structural details of an article in conjunction with NLP methods, e.g., word counts, a "structural" weight can be added to each tag count and be used to predict the role the tag information plays in the storyline. Paragraphs are another document structure with additional information. Through vectorization of articles by paragraphs, additional insight into how groups of tags work together to form the storyline becomes apparent.

2.2.4   One Health Ontology Concept Matching

An ontology is a formal representation of the interrelationships among a set of concepts, terms, and properties within a domain [19]. The One Health Ontology (OHO) is a network of ontologies related to human, animal, and environmental health. OHO concept matching is used to identify terms related to these topics and weigh the probability of the linkage defined. The matching is based on Semantic Resource Description Framework (RDF) graph generation and Web Ontology Language (OWL) description logic reasoning [20]. Through Sematic Web technology stack, NLP concept identification, and graph analytics for concept weighting, key terms relating to biosurveillance are systematically identified and weighted in documents through the Arcturus Framework.

OHO Constitutes. Data with interlinking elements validated across ontologies and quality data curation for the health domain are requirements in ontologies chosen for the OHO [21]. Datasets may contain valuable information, e.g., synonyms for diseases, but lack the required provenance or interlinking elements to validate the additional data into existing classes. The practice of adding elements to an ontology that diverge too far from the original use case domain or removing elements from a merged ontology that are outside of the specific domain should also be avoided.

The existing OHO extends the Pacific Northwest National Laboratory Medical Linked Dataset (PNNL-MLD) [22]. The PNNL-MLD is a composite of well-known medical datasets, e.g., DrugBank (drugbank.ca), Sider (sideeffects.embl.de), PharmGKB (pgrn.org), Pharmacome-diseasome, DailyMed (dailymed.nlm.nih.-gov), DisGeNet (disgenet.org), Wikipedia Infobox (predecessor to WikiData, wikidata.org), and mapped using the Schema.org vocabulary. The OHO extends this dataset to include the Human Disease Ontology (disease-ontology.org), containing the latest research and medical phenomena, as well as updated mappings to the current version of Schema.org. In addition, mappings to disease vectors and locations for current event resolution are included (vectorbase.org). The goal of the final OHO build includes updated instances of emerging pathogens, references to a Gazetter for location resolution, mappings to vectors, and expansions of RDF property relations.

RDF Model. Expressing complex biomedical relationships in a data format that is machine and human readable is accomplished by using the RDF data standard often associated with the Semantic Web [23]. The RDF data model represents ideas as a "triple" of subject-predicate-object expressions, e.g., The *human* (noun) *is infected* (predicate) by the *virus* (object). As these triples are collected and interlinked a large graph of objects and relationships become available to both human researchers and automated machine agents. SPARQL is a query language used to retrieve information from the RDF graphs and the SPARQL query set is what is used to retrieve information from the RDF model [24].

Concept Weight. The concept weight associated with a term is a numerical representation of the confidence that the term identified by the automatic detection algorithm was the object within the OHO. An NER Library generates concept weights by comparing the document to a training library of OHO terms, relationships, and classes of terms. By using the NER term confidence score and averaging it across all scores for the same term within an article, the final value is the concept weight, which is a percentage of certainty that the term exists both within the article and OHO.

Arcturus Framework. Arcturus is a hybrid architecture, within the biosurveillance pipeline, that implements three concurrent stages for streaming data annotation: Data ingestion, NER annotation, and Semantic RDF graph generation and reasoning. The framework is designed to enable expansion of NER algorithms and include new ontologies. The results are stored in an RDF event graph with an internal OWL Event Reporting Ontology for future extensibility in detecting emerging events within a data stream.

Arcturus enables the OHO to become a concept mine within the analytic pipeline, providing speed and accuracy in detecting terms within an article. This functionality is possible through two possible configurations: (1) Query the ontology directly with SPARQL REGEX matching, (2) NER detection with a trained set of tokens and classes mined from an ontology. The 2nd configuration uses the OHO to create a set of training tokens for an NER library. Through a developed set of RDF rules and queries, the OHO is mined for desired terms and synonyms necessary for training the NER library. This library is then used to scan and extract classes of tokens from an English language news feed. Currently, the Arcturus biosurveillance instance assembles selected NER libraries by mining the OHO for core terms, classes, and relationships.

There are many competing technologies that could be combined to form a similar hybrid architecture to Arcturus. The Semantic Web Technology stack is rather limited when including programming libraries, e.g., Apache Jena (jena.apache.org), Redland RDF Libraries (librdf.org), but there are several competing graph databases capable of storing the final event graph [25]. Furthermore, it is not necessary to use a graph database, which are notorious for slow query returns, as small updates to the storage model will create the same semantic graph structure in both relational and key-value data stores without the built-in reasoning capabilities.

2.2.5 Post-processing Algorithm

A post-processing classifier merges features derived from the various extraction methods, i.e., n-gram matching, NER, and Semantic RDF, into a unified labeling schema. This layer of the software system is designed to combine, weight, and encode the respective signals from each method into a user-defined biosurveillance tagging schema (see Sect. 2.2.1). Through this approach, strengths of each methodology are utilized and the final system tags more accurately reflect article elements better than any single method could alone. The post-processing classifier can take many forms depending on the desired tagging schema result and various methods should be tested before a final approach is developed. This is a multi-label document classification problem with a high-quality feature set, i.e., not BoW or simple BoW transformations.

Multi-label document classification is the training and application of many binary classifiers in a process called "Problem Transformation" [26]. Two examples of problem transformations are (1) a new 1/0 classifier is trained for each label that might be applied to a document, i.e., parallel binary relevance (BR), and (2) a new

1/0 classifier is trained for every observed set of labels that has ever been applied to a document, i.e., label power-set binary (PS). These methods represent the extremes of problem transformations for multi-labeled documents. BR does not take advantage of observed co-occurrences of labels, potentially allowing for impossible combinations. PS suffers from a lot of single examples of rare label combinations. Other problem transformations try to bridge the space between BR and PS, while still utilizing a series of 1/0 classifiers, e.g., classifiers for pairs of labels (PL). A review by Madjarov et al. [27] provides an experimental evaluation of choices and explores them in the context of additional methods, such as boosting and applying labels from k Nearest Neighbors [27]. Multi-label document classification is a rich area for research where small modifications of binary relevance can account for dependence of labels [28]. Hierarchy of labels can be represented Directed Acyclic Graphs of label classifiers [29], or in ensembles [30]. Deep-learning with neural networks is an entire different approach, which is promising in large cardinality problems [31, 32].

Despite its simplicity, BR with a strong binary classifier is among the most prominent multi-label text classifier and is used in this pipeline [32]. These final classifiers build on the concepts and/or combination of concepts identified from each of the different tagging processes described above. Since Arcturus is designed to apply only the most relevant tags and n-gram match rules has a high tag label accuracy, this method is appropriate. In addition, the training set did not have any readily discoverable class interactions or mutually exclusive tagging sets. Each post-processing classifier must be trained separately and an empirical distribution function applied to standardize observed feature values.

The input to the algorithm contains all identified features from the pipeline process, e.g., the source method, tag class, tag term/concept, and associated scoring value (i.e., weight or counts). The output is 0/1 if a tag should be applied to a document with n different tags and 2^n combinations of possible tags.

The result of post-processing is a fully normalized output from NLP systems that is indistinguishable from a user-curated document. The primary difference is the shear speed and number of documents that the machine learning system can tag and score compared to a human alone. Future work will incorporate this tagging into event detection and user-interest systems.

References

1. Morrison JP. Flow-based programming. J Appl Dev News. http://ersaconf.org/ersa-adn/papers/adn003.pdf(2013)
2. Eichelberger H, Cui Q, Schmid K (2017) Experiences with the model-based generation of Big Data pipelines. In: conference paper for database systems for business, technology, and the web
3. Hughes JN, Zimmerman MD, Eichelberger CN, Fox AD (2016) A survey of techniques and open-source tools for processing streams of spatio-temporal events. In: Proceedings of the 7th ACM SIGSPATIAL international workshop on GeoStreaming, Article no. 6

4. Stonebraker M, Centitemel U, Zdonik S (2005) The 8 requirements of real-time stream processing. ACM SIGMOD Rec 3(4):42–47
5. Scott S, Matwin S (1999) Feature engineering for text classification. In: Bratko I, Dzeroski S (eds) Proceedings of the sixteenth international conference on machine learning (ICML '99). Morgan Kaufmann Publishers Inc., San Francisco, CA, USA, pp 379–388
6. Shen D, et al (2004, July) Web-page classification through summarization. In: Proceedings of the 27th ACM SIGIR conference on research and development in information retrieval. ACM, pp 242–249
7. Mikolov, T., et al.: Distributed representations of words and phrases and their compositionality. In Advances in neural information processing systems, pp. 3111–3119 (2013)
8. Aggarwal CC, Zhai CX (2012) A survey of text classification algorithms. In: Mining text data, pp 163–222
9. Hastie T, et al (2008) The Elements of statistical learning, 2nd edn. Springer. ISBN 0-387-95284-5
10. Robertson S (2004) Understanding inverse document frequency: on theoretical arguments for IDF. J Doc 60(5):503–520
11. Chang M, Yih W, Meek C (2008) Partitioned logistic regression for spam filtering. In: Proceedings of the 14th ACM SIGKDD International Conference on Knowledge Discovery and Data Mining (KDD '08). ACM, New York, NY, USA, pp 97–105
12. Blei D, Lafferty J (2009) Topic models. In: Srivastava A, Sahami M (eds) Text mining: theory and applications. Taylor and Francis
13. Stoddard G (2015) Popularity and quality in social news aggregators: a study of reddit and hacker news. In: Proceedings of the 24th International Conference on World Wide Web. ACM
14. Fellbaum C (ed) (1998) WordNet: an electronic lexical database. MIT Press, Cambridge, MA
15. Manning CD et al (2014, June) The Stanford CoreNLP natural language processing toolkit. In: ACL (System Demonstrations), pp 55–60
16. Bird S, Klein E, Loper E (2009) Natural language processing with python—analyzing text with the natural language toolkit. O'reilly Media. www.nltk.org
17. Hochreiter S, Schmidhuber J (1997) Long short-term memory. Neural Comput 9(8):1735–1780
18. Toutanova K, Klein D, Manning CD, Singer Y (2003) Feature-rich part-of-speech tagging with a cyclic dependency network. In: Proceedings of the 2003 Conference of the North American Chapter of the Association for Computational Linguistics on Human Language Technology, vol 1, pp 252–259
19. Arp R, Smith B, Spear AD (2016) Building ontologies with basic formal ontology. MIT Press, 248 pp
20. Baader F, et al (2003) The description logic handbook: theory, implementation and applications. Cambridge University Press, 555 pp
21. Bizer C, Heath T, Berners-Lee T (2009) Linked data-the story so far. In: Semantic services, interoperability and web applications: emerging concepts, pp 205–227
22. Smith W, Chappell A, Corley C (April 2015) Medical and transmission vector vocabulary alignment with Schema. org. In: International Conference on Biomedical Ontology (ICBO); Buffalo, NY
23. Berners-Lee T, Hendler J, Lassila O (2001) The Semantic web. Sci Am 284(5):28–37
24. Prud'hommeaux E, Seaborne A (2006) SPARQL query language for RDF
25. Nitta K, Savnik I (2014) Survey of RDF storage managers. In: Proceedings of the 6th international conference on advances in databases, knowledge, and data applications (DBKDA'14), Chamonix, France, pp 148–153
26. Read J, Pfahringer B, Holmes G (2008) Multi-label classification using ensembles of pruned sets. Data Mining. In: IEEE International Conference on ICDM'08. Eighth. IEEE
27. Madjarov G et al (2012) An extensive experimental comparison of methods for multi-label learning. Pattern Recogn 45(9):3084–3104

28. Montañes E et al (2014) Dependent binary relevance models for multi-label classification. Pattern Recogn 47(3):1494–1508

29. Gibaja E, Sebastián V (2014) Multi-label learning: a review of the state of the art and ongoing research. Wiley Interdisc Rev Data Min Knowl Discov 4(6):411–444

30. Zhang L, Shah SK, Kakadiaris IA (2017) Hierarchical multi-label classification using fully associative ensemble learning. Pattern Recogn 70:89–103

31. Liu J et al (2017, August) Deep learning for extreme multi-label text classification. In: Proceedings of the 40th ACM SIGIR conference on research and development in information retrieval. ACM, pp 115–124

32. Nam J et al (2014) Large-scale multi-label text classification—revisiting neural networks. In: Joint European conference on machine learning and knowledge discovery in databases. Springer, Berlin, Heidelberg

Cited Software

33. Amazon Web Services Lambda. https://aws.amazon.com/lambda/
34. Apache Flink. https://flink.apache.org/
35. Apache Jena. https://jena.apache.org/
36. Apache Kafka. https://kafka.apache.org/
37. Apache NIFI. https://nifi.apache.org/
38. Apache Lucene. https://lucene.apache.org/
39. Apache Storm. http://storm.apache.org/
40. ElasticSearch. https://www.elastic.co/
41. MITIE. https://github.com/mit-nlp/MITIE
42. MongoDB. https://www.mongodb.com/
43. Redland RDF. http://librdf.org/
44. Spark. https://spark.apache.org/
45. WordNet. https://wordnet.princeton.edu/
46. Python Goose. https://github.com/grangier/python-goose
47. Python natural language tool kit. http://www.nltk.org/
48. Python newspaper. http://newspaper.readthedocs.io/
49. Stanford CoreNLP. https://stanfordnlp.github.io/CoreNLP/index.html
50. Word2Vec. https://code.google.com/archive/p/word2vec/

Part IV
Case Studies

Young Adults, Health Insurance Expansions and Hospital Services Utilization

Teresa B. Gibson, Zeynal Karaca, Gary Pickens, Michael Dworsky, Eli Cutler, Brian J. Moore, Richele Benevent and Herbert Wong

Abstract Under the dependent coverage expansion (DCE) provision of health reform adult children up to 26 years of age whose parents have employer-sponsored or individual health insurance are eligible for insurance under their parents' health plan. Using a difference-in-differences approach and the 2008–2014 Healthcare Cost and Utilization Project State Emergency Department Databases and State Inpatient Databases we examined the impact of the DCE on hospital services use. In analyses of individuals age <26 years (compared to individuals over 26) we found a 1.5% increase in non-pregnancy related inpatient visits in 2010 through 2013 during the initial DCE period and a 1.6% increase in 2014 when other state expansions went into effect. We found that the impact of the DCE persisted into 2014 when many state insurance expansions occurred, although effects varied for states adopting and not adopting Medicaid expansions.

1 Introduction

One of the first provisions of the Affordable Care Act to take effect was an expansion of insurance coverage for young adults up to 26 years of age whose parents have employer-sponsored or individual health insurance. This provision applied to all new plan years starting on or after September 23, 2010—as of that date, adult children, regardless of residence, student status, or marital status, were

T. B. Gibson (✉) · G. Pickens · E. Cutler · B. J. Moore · R. Benevent
Truven Health Analytics, 100 Phoenix Dr., Ann Arbor, MI 48108, USA
e-mail: teresa.gibson@us.ibm.com

Z. Karaca · H. Wong
Agency for Health Services Research and Quality, Bethesda, MD, USA

M. Dworsky
RAND, Santa Monica, CA, USA

© Springer International Publishing AG, part of Springer Nature 2018   135
P. J. Giabbanelli et al. (eds.), *Advanced Data Analytics in Health*, Smart Innovation,
Systems and Technologies 93, https://doi.org/10.1007/978-3-319-77911-9_8

eligible for insurance under their parents' health plan [35]. This eligibility under their parents' health plan was extended to young adults regardless of whether they were eligible for insurance through another employer or through a state insurance exchange. Prior to the dependent care coverage expansion (DCE), young adults had the highest rates of uninsurance of any age group [11] and low rates of access to employment-based insurance [35].

In 2014 health insurance choices for the young adult age group expanded further with all states offering coverage through Health Insurance Exchanges (HIX) and through Medicaid expansions in certain states. The DCE remains in effect, allowing young adults to opt for coverage under their parents' health insurance plan. In this study we investigate the impact of the dependent care coverage expansion enacted in 2010 that provides health insurance to young adults and the impact of the expansion on ED and inpatient visits through 2014.

A great deal of evidence has been produced about the impact of the DCE [8, 14], focusing on a wide variety of impacts such as shifts in coverage patterns [2, 12, 21, 32, 33], declines in uninsurance, disparities in the impact of the DCE [9, 16, 21, 26] and other impacts on outcomes or use [7, 10, 22, 31, 38, 4, 29, 31]. Many focus on the DCE impact within subgroups such as individuals with mental illness [1, 20], cystic fibrosis [33], substance use disorder [30], and cancer [2, 17, 27]. While a few studies address utilization patterns, and find shifts to privately insured visits and away from uninsured visits, there is little evidence on how utilization among young adults targeted by the DCE has evolved over time.

Our study adds to the literature by analyzing inpatient utilization using HCUP data from 36 states and ED utilization from 19 states in 2008–2014. We estimate the DCE impact in 2Q2010-2013, the initial time period after the DCE was implemented, and in 2014, after the private and state Medicaid insurance expansions. To our knowledge, ours if the first study that includes the 2014 time period, when major Medicaid expansions occurred in a large number of states, expanding the eligibility for the Medicaid program within participating states so more individuals could be eligible for coverage. We examine the impact of the DCE during this important time period in two ways to determine if the impact of the DCE policy persisted. First, we isolate the DCE impact within expansion states and within nonexpansion states separately to see if the DCE impact is different. Second, we estimate the 2014 DCE impact for all states combined to analyse the average impact. We use a difference-in-differences framework, comparing the experiences of young adults eligible for the DCE to a comparison group slightly older in age but not eligible for the DCE and answer the following research questions.

1. What was the impact of the DCE on hospital services utilization patterns prior to the state insurance expansions and after the expansions?
2. Was the impact on young adults different in expansion and non-expansion states?

2 Methods

Our primary data source was the all-payer HCUP State Inpatient Databases (SID) and State Emergency Department Databases (SEDD) from 2008 through 2014. Hospital inpatient discharge and ED records were assembled from the HCUP SID and SEDD and our sample included 2008–2014 SID data from 36 states —18 expansion states and 18 non-expansion states. We included 2008–2014 SEDD data for 19 states—9 expansion states and 10 non-expansion states. Discharges and visits for community, non-rehabilitation hospitals as defined in the American Hospital Association Annual Survey were included.

The SID used for the study were Arizona, Arkansas, California, Colorado, Connecticut, Florida, Georgia, Hawaii, Illinois, Indiana, Iowa, Kansas, Kentucky, Louisiana, Minnesota, Missouri, Nebraska, Nevada, New Jersey, New York, North Carolina, Ohio, Oklahoma, Oregon, Pennsylvania, Rhode Island, South Carolina, South Dakota, Tennessee, Texas, Utah, Virginia, Washington, West Virginia, Wisconsin, Wyoming. The SEDD used for the study were California, Connecticut, Florida, Georgia, Indiana, Iowa, Kansas, Kentucky, Minnesota, Missouri, Nebraska, New Jersey, New York, North Carolina, Ohio, Rhode Island, South Carolina, Tennessee, and Wisconsin.

ED and inpatient nonpregnancy visits were counted by state, calendar quarter, primary payer, gender, and year of age (or age cohort) throughout the study time period. We used population estimates from the U.S. Census Bureau by state, year, gender, and age to construct ED and inpatient visit rates per quarter, by applying the population counts to each quarter of the year. We counted mental health visits that require hospitalization in young adults defined using Clinical Classifications Software (CCS) categories. We also included indicators for several ambulatory-sensitive conditions defined using the AHRQ Prevention Quality Indicators [37], suggesting that care may not have been well-delivered in the ambulatory setting (asthma for inpatient and ED visits, bacterial pneumonia for inpatient discharges, and a composite measure (PQI 90) for inpatient discharges).

Our estimation framework compares the experiences of young adults exposed to the policy change (age 20–25) to an older age group (age 27–33) using a difference-in-differences framework to detect changes in trends associated with the DCE, an approach similar to most studies addressing the impact of the DCE [8]. We do not include 19 and 26 year olds due to mixed eligibility for the DCE within a year [35]. A common assumption with the difference-in-differences approach is that the intervention and comparison groups follow similar pre-intervention trends which allows us to detect differences trends following the DCE while controlling for observable differences. We performed a test of pre-period equivalence in trends for the intervention and comparison groups, and found statistical equivalence in all outcomes except private asthma ED visits, and inpatient total and mental health discharges for private pay and uninsured. In these cases, trend differences were small in magnitude. We excluded pregnancy visits due to differences in pre-period trends.

Population characteristics for each state at the state-age-gender-year level were obtained for all individuals and by payer from the one-year U.S. Census Bureau American Community Survey Integrated Public Use Microdata Samples (IPUMS). These characteristics included marital status, household income, education, employment status, race, and ethnicity [34]. We also calculated the percentage of the population living with parents and the percentage employed full time from the IPUMS) [28].

Our estimation framework relies on age, state, and time fixed effects to isolate variation in policy exposure at a given age across states. We estimate the change in rates of each event (ED visit or inpatient discharge) per population associated with contemporaneous exposure to the dependent care expansion and the Medicaid/HIX expansions using generalized linear models with state and time fixed effects with the following specification for the conditional mean of the utilization rate.

$$
\begin{aligned}
E(Y_{ast}|X, a, s, t) = \exp(&\alpha_0 + \alpha_1 DCE_t * AgeGroup_a + \alpha_2 ME_{st} + \alpha_3(ME_{st} = 0) * AgeGroup_a \\
&+ \alpha_4(ME_{st} = 1) * AgeGroup_a + X_{ast}\alpha_5 + \alpha_6 female_{ast} + \mu_a + \pi_t + \theta_s
\end{aligned}
$$

$$(1)$$

In this specification, Y_{ast} is defined as the count of ED or inpatient visits for individuals of age a (in single-year increments) in state s at time t (in calendar quarters). The population count for each state, calendar quarter, and age is specified as the offset term, which is omitted from the equation for simplicity. AgeGroup = 1 if the individual was age 20–25 years and 0 if 27–33 years. DCE is a dummy data element that equals 1 in the ACA dependent coverage expansion period (third quarter 2010 through fourth quarter 2013) and 0 otherwise. We start with the second quarter of 2010 as employers were permitted to implement the DCE immediately [36]. ME is also an indicator variable, equal to 1 if state s expanded Medicaid in 2014, 0 otherwise. Fixed effects for age (μ_a), time (π_t), and state (θ_s) are included and absorb the uninteracted effects for AgeGroup, DCE, and ACA. X_{ast} includes control variables such as measures of labor market conditions and cell average demographics, and we include an indicator for female gender. Age effects control for the long-run average age profile of utilization; time dummies account for secular trends; and state effects control for time-invariant, state-specific factors.

The interaction AgeGroup * DCE provides the proportionate difference-in-differences estimate of the contemporaneous impact of the DCE policy. Exponentiated coefficients [e.g., $\exp(\alpha_1)$], less 1, represent the adjusted percentage change in utilization rates associated with the insurance expansions. We create two interaction terms (MEst = 0) * AgeGroup and (MEst = 1) * AgeGroup to allow us to examine the 2014 DCE impact in expansion states and in non-expansion states where MEst = 1 in states with a Medicaid expansion in effect in 2014. Accordingly, the term (ME_st = 1) * AgeGroup compares 2014 experiences for under 26 year olds in expansion states to over 26 year olds in expansion states to isolate the DCE impact in these states. Likewise, the term (ME_st = 0) * AgeGroup compares 2014 experiences for under 26 year olds in nonexpansion states to over 26 year olds in nonexpansion states.

We then modify the specification and estimate the DCE impact for all states combined in 2014 (without a differentiation for expansion status, (Post_2014 = 1 in 2014), with the over 26 year old group in both groups of states serving as a comparison group for the under 26 year old group in both groups of states.

$$E(Y_{ast}|X, a, s, t) = \exp(\beta_0 + \beta_1 DCE_t * AgeGroup_a + \beta_2 ME_{st} + \beta_3 Post\_2014 * AgeGroup_a$$
$$+ X_{ast}\beta_4 + \beta_5 female_{ast} + \mu_a + \pi_t + \theta_s$$

$$(2)$$

3 Results

ED data originated from 19 states that participated in both the SID and SEDD from 2008 through 2014, representing 13.9 million young adults less than 26 years of age annually and 15.4 million young adults in the comparison group over age 26 (see Table 1). Inpatient discharge data originated from 36 SID states representing 22.6 million young adults under age 26 annually and 25.1 million over age 26. The population of young adults eligible for the dependent care insurance coverage expansion and those in the comparison group were similar in terms of demographic characteristics prior to the DCE, including percentage female, racial composition, and ethnic composition. These young adults differed from the comparison group in socioeconomic characteristics such as college graduation rates (15.8% for those under age 26 and 32% for those older than 26) (not shown) and living with parents (41.3% for those under age 26 and 14.4% for those older than 26), as expected.

ED visit rates were 9,737 per 100,000 population per quarter in the under 26 age group and 9,327 per 100,000 population for those older than age 26. Inpatient discharge rates were 748 per 100,000 population per quarter in the under age 26 group and 993 per 100,000 population for the group over age 26.

When analyzing the impact of the dependent care coverage expansion to age 26 years in 2Q2010-2013, we found that the policy change was associated with an increase in inpatient discharges (1.5% higher, $p < 0.01$, see Table 2). In 2014, after

Table 1 Population characteristics, emergency department visit rates and inpatient discharge rates per 100,000 Population (2008–2009)

Variable	Characteristics with emergency department data				Characteristics with inpatient discharge data			
	<26 years		>26 years		<26 years		>26 years	
No. of states	19		19		36		36	
Population count (total in 000 s)	13,901		15,364		22,585		25,109	
	Mean (%)	SD	Mean (%)	SD	Mean (%)	SD	Mean (%)	SD
% Female	48.8	0.500	49.8	0.500	48.7	0.500	49.7	0.500
% Married	13.4	0.089	46.1	0.096	14.5	0.096	47.3	0.096
Household income (%)								
<$35,000	32.2	0.079	25.5	0.063	32.7	0.074	25.6	0.061
$35,000–$75,000	31.6	0.050	35.8	0.049	31.7	0.052	36.3	0.046
>$75,000	30.0	0.087	36.4	0.094	29.4	0.079	35.7	0.085
% Lives with parents	41.3	0.115	14.4	0.056	39.8	0.114	13.8	0.054
Race (%)								
White	70.9	0.098	70.8	0.103	72.5	0.094	72.7	0.097
Black or African American	15.7	0.082	14.3	0.078	14.8	0.082	13.2	0.076
Other	13.4	0.103	14.9	0.108	12.7	0.089	14.1	0.093
Ethnicity								
Hispanic	21.1	0.149	21.4	0.141	21.6	0.147	21.9	0.139
Medicaid expansion state	57.2	0.495	57.9	0.494	51.3	0.500	52.2	0.500
Visit and discharge rates per 100,000 population per quarter[a]	Emergency department data				Inpatient discharge data			
	<26 years		>26 years		<26 years		>26 years	
	Mean	SD	Mean	SD	Mean	SD	Mean	SD
Total[a]	9,737	3,540	9,327	3,205	748	181	993	254
Condition								
Mental health	1,726	1,136	1,905	1,175	411	169	561	205
Asthma	392	192	458	236	9	8	14	10
Bacterial pneumonia	N/A	N/A	N/A	N/A	10	7	15	9
Overall PQI	N/A	N/A	N/A	N/A	65	33	88	34
Primary payer[a]								
Uninsured	2,923	2,454	2,360	1,861	220	112	257	138
Private insurance	3,467	1,422	3,445	1,336	296	90	392	130
Medicaid	3,565	1,889	3,172	1,520	156	87	192	88

Data Source The SID used for the study were Arizona, Arkansas, California, Colorado, Connecticut, Florida, Georgia, Hawaii, Illinois, Indiana, Iowa, Kansas, Kentucky, Louisiana, Minnesota, Missouri, Nebraska, Nevada, New Jersey, New York, North Carolina, Ohio, Oklahoma, Oregon, Pennsylvania, Rhode Island, South Carolina, South Dakota, Tennessee, Texas, Utah, Virginia, Washington, West Virginia, Wisconsin, Wyoming. The SEDD used for the study were California, Connecticut, Florida, Georgia, Indiana, Iowa, Kansas, Kentucky, Minnesota, Missouri, Nebraska, New Jersey, New York, North Carolina, Ohio, Rhode Island, South Carolina, Tennessee, and Wisconsin
[a]non-pregnancy
Labor Force participation and educational attainment not included

Table 2 Impact of the dependent care insurance expansion, inpatient discharges

	3Q2010–2013		All States 2013–2014		Expansion states[a] 2013–2014		Non-expansion states[a] 2013–2014	
	Change in rate (%)	95% CI	Change in rate (%)	95% CI	Change in rate (%)	95% CI	Change in rate (%)	95% CI
All payer inpatient discharges								
Total[b]	0.015***	(0.008, 0.021)	0.016***	(0.006, 0.027)	0.041***	(0.026, 0.055)	−0.008	(−0.022, 0.006)
Mental health	0.003	(−0.005, 0.010)	0.024***	(0.013, 0.036)	0.041***	(0.025, 0.056)	0.007	(−0.008, 0.023)
Asthma	0.026*	(−0.002, 0.054)	0.013	(−0.034, 0.062)	0.086***	(0.021, 0.156)	−0.061*	(−0.121, 0.002)
Bacterial pneumonia	−0.049***	(−0.073, −0.025)	−0.052**	(−0.094, −0.007)	−0.017	(−0.078, 0.048)	−0.082***	(−0.137, −0.023)
Total PQI	0.025***	(0.012, 0.038)	0.030***	(0.009, 0.052)	0.076***	(0.045, 0.107)	−0.009	(−0.036, 0.019)
Medicaid inpatient discharges								
Total[b]	−0.102***	(−0.113, −0.090)	−0.016*	(−0.035, 0.003)	−0.010	(−0.032, 0.012)	−0.027*	(−0.055, 0.002)
Mental Health	−0.097***	(−0.110, −0.083)	−0.020*	(−0.040, 0.000)	−0.037***	(−0.060, −0.012)	0.009	(−0.020, 0.040)
Asthma	−0.103***	(−0.144, −0.061)	0.032	(−0.041, 0.110)	0.136***	(0.042, 0.237)	−0.144**	(−0.240, −0.036)
Bacterial Pneumonia	−0.155***	(−0.192, −0.116)	−0.111***	(−0.177, −0.039)	−0.065	(−0.150, 0.028)	−0.175***	(−0.267, −0.073)
Total PQI	−0.052***	(−0.073, −0.031)	0.014	(−0.02, 0.049)	0.052**	(0.009, 0.096)	−0.040	(−0.088, 0.010)
Private inpatient discharges								
Total[b]	0.265***	(0.254, 0.277)	0.129***	(0.112, 0.146)	0.173***	(0.150, 0.197)	0.088***	(0.066, 0.110)
Mental health	0.274***	(0.260, 0.289)	0.104***	(0.086, 0.123)	0.119***	(0.094, 0.144)	0.091***	(0.066, 0.115)
Asthma	0.284***	(0.225, 0.347)	0.134***	(0.045, 0.231)	0.262***	(0.133, 0.406)	0.009	(−0.100, 0.132)
Bacterial pneumonia	0.157***	(0.110, 0.206)	0.035	(−0.040, 0.117)	0.067	(−0.040, 0.187)	0.009	(−0.086, 0.114)
Total PQI	0.285***	(0.260, 0.311)	0.159***	(0.122, 0.197)	0.226***	(0.173, 0.282)	0.102***	(0.056, 0.150)

(continued)

Table 2 (continued)

	3Q2010-2013		All States 2013–2014		Expansion states[a] 2013–2014		Non-expansion states[a] 2013–2014	
	Change in rate (%)	95% CI	Change in rate (%)	95% CI	Change in rate (%)	95% CI	Change in rate (%)	95% CI
Uninsured inpatient discharges								
Total[b]	-0.143***	(-0.154, -0.132)	-0.078***	(-0.099, -0.055)	-0.047**	(-0.082, -0.010)	-0.095***	(-0.117, -0.073)
Mental health	-0.152***	(-0.164, -0.139)	-0.051***	(-0.076, -0.026)	0.017	(-0.025, 0.061)	-0.082***	(-0.106, -0.058)
Asthma	-0.044*	(-0.089, 0.004)	-0.048	(-0.132, 0.044)	0.021	(-0.131, 0.199)	-0.077	(-0.171, 0.027)
Bacterial pneumonia	-0.147***	(-0.189, -0.104)	-0.092*	(-0.179, 0.004)	0.063	(-0.109, 0.269)	-0.153***	(-0.247, -0.048)
Total PQI	-0.089***	(-0.110, -0.067)	-0.041*	(-0.082, 0.001)	-0.019	(-0.097, 0.065)	-0.059***	(-0.102, -0.014)

[a]All States; Comparison group consists of all individuals over age 26 in all states

Expansion States: Comparison group consists of all individuals over age 26 in expansion states

Non Expansion States: Comparison group consists of all individuals over age 26 in non-expansion states

[b]Nonpregnancy related totals

***, **, *$p \leq 0.01$, **$0.01 < p \leq 0.05$, *$0.05 < p \leq 0.10$

the state expansions, the total discharge rate increased 1.6% for the DCE-eligible group relative to the comparison group.

Medicaid discharge rates declined in the DCE period (2Q2010-2013) with most reductions exceeding 9%. Medicaid discharge rates also declined in 2014, but to a lesser degree. In the DCE period private pay discharges for all conditions rose, and in 2014, private pay discharge rates increased at a smaller magnitude.

In both time periods, rates of uninsured discharges declined in the DCE time period, with most reductions exceeding 14%. In 2014, the magnitude of the drop was smaller, with relative rates of uninsured discharges (relative to rates in the over 26 group) smaller than a 10% decrease.

When examining the change in discharges from 2013 to 2014 relative to the over age 26 group in similar (non-expansion or expansion) states we found that rates of non-pregnancy related discharges were 4.1% higher in expansion states and no different than the comparison group in non-expansion states. Private discharges for the DCE eligible group in expansion states were 17.3% higher than the comparison group for total non-pregnancy related discharges. In non-expansion states private discharges increased to a lesser degree, 8.8%.

Uninsured non-pregnancy related discharges decreased to a similar degree in expansion and non-expansion states (4.7% and 9.5% respectively).

Many trends for ED visits mirrored those described above for inpatient discharges with increases in private pay visits across all time periods (see Table 3). There was a shift away from Medicaid in the early DCE period, which continued in 2014 in non-expansion states.

In addition, we acknowledge that when relying on contemporaneous age there may be some cross-contamination of the intervention and comparison groups as those originally in the intervention group age out. We performed a sensitivity analysis, focusing on a comparison of 20–23 year olds with 29–30 year olds, and found no significant difference in results. A sensitivity analysis with a comparison group of 27–29 year olds who may be more similar to the intervention group was similar to the reported results.

4 Discussion

In this study, we estimated the effects of the dependent care coverage expansion on ED and inpatient visits through 2014, extending the literature into the fourth year after policy implementation, which has been, to our knowledge, unexplored in the literature [3, 5, 6, 8, 14, 23]. Major trends in the DCE time period were a shift toward private visits and discharges, a shift away from Medicaid visits and discharges, and significantly lower rates of uninsured visits and discharges. These

Table 3 Impact of the dependent care insurance expansion, emergency department visits

	3Q2010-2013		All States 2013-2014		Expansion states[a] 2013-2014		Non-expansion states[a] 2013-2014	
	Change in rate (%)	95% CI	Change in rate (%)	95% CI	Change in rate (%)	95% CI	Change in rate (%)	95% CI
All payer emergency department visits								
Total[b]	-0.036***	(-0.041, -0.031)	-0.005	(-0.012, 0.003)	0.009*	(-0.001, 0.019)	-0.020***	(-0.031, -0.009)
Mental health	-0.057***	(-0.064, -0.051)	-0.003	(-0.012, 0.006)	0.022***	(0.009, 0.035)	-0.028***	(-0.04, -0.015)
Asthma	0.016***	(0.006, 0.027)	0.008	(-0.008, 0.024)	0.013	(-0.007, 0.033)	0.000	(-0.023, 0.024)
Medicaid emergency department visits								
Total[b]	-0.109***	(-0.121, -0.096)	-0.026***	(-0.045, -0.008)	-0.006	(-0.028, 0.016)	-0.056***	(-0.084, -0.029)
Mental health	-0.131***	(-0.145, -0.118)	-0.028***	(-0.046, -0.009)	-0.002	(-0.024, 0.02)	-0.060***	(-0.085, -0.034)
Asthma	-0.051***	(-0.071, -0.031)	0.013	(-0.015, 0.042)	0.039**	(0.006, 0.073)	-0.046*	(-0.09, 0.001)
Private emergency department visits								
Total[b]	0.158***	(0.150, 0.167)	0.091***	(0.079, 0.103)	0.110***	(0.094, 0.125)	0.066***	(0.049, 0.084)
Mental Health	0.232***	(0.219, 0.245)	0.112***	(0.097, 0.128)	0.152***	(0.132, 0.173)	0.067***	(0.047, 0.088)
Asthma	0.246***	(0.224, 0.268)	0.139***	(0.108, 0.172)	0.140***	(0.102, 0.18)	0.142***	(0.095, 0.191)
Uninsured emergency department visits								
Total[b]	-0.114***	(-0.122, -0.107)	-0.037***	(-0.051, -0.023)	-0.005	(-0.026, 0.017)	-0.059***	(-0.075, -0.043)
Mental health	-0.134***	(-0.143, -0.124)	-0.026***	(-0.042, -0.011)	0.051***	(0.025, 0.077)	-0.065***	(-0.081, -0.048)
Asthma	-0.063***	(-0.078, -0.048)	-0.036***	(-0.062, -0.01)	0.003	(-0.036, 0.042)	-0.063***	(-0.094, -0.032)

[a]All States; Comparison group consists of all individuals over age 26 in all states

Expansion States: Comparison group consists of all individuals over age 26 in expansion states

Non Expansion States: Comparison group consists of all individuals over age 26 in non-expansion states

[b]Nonpregnancy related totals

*** $p \leq 0.01$, ** $0.01 < p \leq 0.05$, * $0.05 < p \leq 0.10$

results are consistent with those from other studies [24] Inpatient visits (non-pregnancy) increased subsequent to the coverage expansion. We also found that the dependent care coverage expansion increased access to inpatient care for young adults. These results are consistent with findings from quasi-experimental studies evaluating the Affordable Care Act dependent care coverage expansion on mental health inpatient admissions from California, Florida, and New York [18, 15]. It is also consistent with earlier findings from Anderson et al. [3], who evaluated the effects of losing health insurance coverage at age 19 because of exclusion from parental health insurance plans, as well as with analyses of Medicaid expansions during the mid-1980s and early 1990s [13], and recent findings reported by Antwi et al. [5].

We found small declines in ED use after DCE implementation, a result consistent with the findings of Hernandez-Boussard and colleagues [19]. We also found a shift to privately insured visits, and away from Medicaid and uninsured visits, a result that was also consistent with Hernandez-Boussard (2016).

These trends shifted after the state expansions in 2014. Expansion states experienced much higher adjusted utilization rates for Medicaid visits and discharges, and large declines in uninsured. The DCE impact on private insurance appeared to have persisted into 2014, as evidenced by higher rates of private insurance utilization for DCE-exposed cohorts relative to comparison cohorts, albeit at a somewhat lower rate relative to the initial DCE time frame. The smaller impact of the DCE may originate from increased access to other sources of private insurance from the exchanges for all age groups, and increased access to Medicaid in expansion states.

Our study has several limitations. We lacked an untreated comparison group of the same age due to the national reach of the DCE. Like other studies addressing DCE impacts, the comparison group we used was older than the intervention group, with differences in labor market and sociodemographic characteristics. However, we performed a sensitivity analysis narrowing the age group of the comparison group to 27–29 years of age and our results were similar. Our approach is based on the assumption that the trends in the intervention group would have been similar those in the comparison group (those not eligible for the DCE). Another assumption is that the changes in 2014 (health insurance exchanges and Medicaid expansions) had the same impact on the intervention and comparison group. If these are not the case, then this could bias our results. In addition, we could not follow individuals over time. Future studies involving data sources tracking individuals and their families should analyse the impact of the DCE on those who were targeted by the policy: uninsured young adults with privately-insured parents. On a related note, other programs, either local expansions or firms that extended coverage to young adults may have been in effect prior to the DCE, and we were unable to account for these programs. Therefore, our effects should be interpreted as population-level averages incremental to any existing programs. Finally, our data includes hospital services and the impact of the DCE may differ in other settings. These patterns also suggest that own-price effects dominate with insurance, and care should be exercised when populations are offered coverage to minimize inappropriate use. However, insurance coverage may also lead to more medically indicated admissions—for example, access to nursing call-in lines that can help patients decide whether their condition warrants a hospital or ED visit could either increase or decrease admissions depending on the patient's reported symptoms [25]. Although we report primarily on trends in utilization by payer and condition, we do not have information on the appropriateness of these services.

5   Conclusions

These results confirm that the dependent care coverage expansion was working as intended by significantly relieving the payment burden for a large number of young adults and likely improving the financial condition of EDs and hospitals that typically collect less from uninsured patients. In analyses of individuals age 20–25 who were in the DCE-eligible age range compared to individuals age 27–33 we found a 1.5% increase in non-pregnancy related inpatient visits and a 3.6% decrease in non-pregnancy related emergency department visits in 2010 through 2013 during the initial DCE period. We also found that the impact of the DCE persisted into 2014 when many state insurance expansions occurred, although effects varied for states adopting and not adopting Medicaid expansions.

Acknowledgements This study was funded by the Agency for Healthcare Research and Quality under contract HHSA-290-2013-00002-C. The views expressed herein are those of the authors and do not necessarily reflect those of the Agency for Healthcare Research and Quality or the U.S. Department of Health and Human Services. No official endorsement by any agency of the federal or state governments, Truven Health Analytics or RAND Corporation is intended or should be inferred. No potential conflicts of interest exist.

The authors would like to acknowledge the following HCUP Partner organizations for contributing data to the HCUP State Inpatient Databases (SID) used in this study: Arizona, Arkansas, California, Colorado, Connecticut, Florida, Georgia, Hawaii, Illinois, Indiana, Iowa, Kansas, Kentucky, Louisiana, Minnesota, Missouri, Nebraska, Nevada, New Jersey, New York, North Carolina, Ohio, Oklahoma, Oregon, Pennsylvania, Rhode Island, South Carolina, South Dakota, Tennessee, Texas, Utah, Virginia, Washington, West Virginia, Wisconsin, Wyoming. The authors would also like to acknowledge the following HCUP Partner organizations for contributing data to the HCUP State Emergency Department Databases (SEDD) used in this study: California, Connecticut, Florida, Georgia, Indiana, Iowa, Kansas, Kentucky, Minnesota, Missouri, Nebraska, New Jersey, New York, North Carolina, Ohio, Rhode Island, South Carolina, Tennessee, Wisconsin. A full list of HCUP Data Partners can be found at www.hcup-us.ahrq.gov/hcupdatapartners.jsp.

References

1. Ali MM, Chen J, Mutter R, Novak P, Mortensen K (2016) The ACA's Dependent Coverage Expansion and Out-of-Pocket Spending by Young Adults With Behavioral Health Conditions. Psychiatr Serv 67(9):977–982
2. Alvarez EM, Keegan T, Johnston EE, Haile R, Sanders L, Wise P (2017) The affordable care act dependent coverage expansion (ACA-DCE): disparities in impact in young adult oncology patients. J Clin Oncol 35(15):6561
3. Anderson M, Dobkin C, Gross T (2012) The effect of health insurance coverage on the use of medical services. Am Econ J Econ Policy 4(1):1–27
4. Antwi YA, Moriya AS, Simon K (2012) Effects of federal policy to insure young adults: evidence from the 2010 Affordable Care Act dependent coverage mandate. NBER Working Paper No.18200. http://www.nber.org/papers/w18200
5. Antwi YA, Moriya AS, Simon K, Sommers BD (2015) Changes in emergency department use among young adults after the patient protection and affordable care act's dependent coverage provision. Ann Emerg Med 65(6):664–672
6. Antwi YA, Moriya AS, Simon K (2015) Access to health insurance and the use of inpatient medical care: evidence from the affordable care act young adult mandate. J Health Econ 39 (2015):171–187
7. Barbaresco S, Courtemanche CJ, Qi Y (2015) Impacts of the affordable care act dependent coverage provision on health-related outcomes of young adults. J Health Econ 40:54–68
8. Breslau J, Stein BD, Han B, Shelton S, Yu H (2018) Impact of the affordable care act's dependent coverage expansion on the health care and health status of young adults. Med Care Res Rev 75(2):131–152
9. Breslau J, Han B, Stein BD, Burns RM, Yu H (2017) Did the affordable care act's dependent coverage expansion affect race/ethnic disparities in health insurance coverage? Health Serv Res. https://doi.org/10.1111/1475-6773.12728
10. Busch SH, Golberstein E, Meara E (2014) ACA dependent coverage provision reduced high out-of-pocket health care spending for young adults. Health Aff 33(8):1361–1366
11. Collins SR, Robertson R, Garber T, Doty MM (2013) Insuring the future: Current trends in health coverage and the effects of implementing the Affordable Care Act. The Commonwealth Fund. http://www.commonwealthfund.org/Publications/Fund-Reports/2013/Apr/Insuring-the-Future.aspx
12. Courtemanche C, Marton J, Ukert B, Yelowitz A, Zapata D (2016) Impacts of the affordable care act on health insurance coverage in medicaid expansion and non-expansion states. NBER Working paper 22182. www.nber.org
13. Currie J, Gruber J (1996) Health insurance eligibility, utilization of medical care, and child health. Q J Econ 111(2):431–466
14. French MT, Homer J, Gumus G, Hickling L (2016) Key provisions of the patient protection and affordable care act (ACA): a systematic review and presentation of early research findings. Health Serv Res 51(5):1735–1771
15. Golberstein E, Busch SH, Zaha R, Greenfield SF, Beardslee WR, Meara E (2015) Effect of the affordable care act's young adult insurance expansions on hospital-based mental health care. Am J Psychiatry 172(2):182–189. https://doi.org/10.1176/appi.ajp.2014.14030375
16. Han X, Zhu S, Jemal A (2016) Characteristics of young adults enrolled through the affordable care act-dependent coverage expansion. J Adolesc Health 59(6):648–653
17. Han X, Zang Xiong K, Kramer MR, Jemal A (2016) The affordable care act and cancer stage at diagnosis among young adults. J Natl Cancer Inst 108(9)
18. Hernandez-Boussard T, Burns CS, Ewen Wang N, Baker LC, Goldstein BA (2014) The affordable care act reduces emergency department use by young adults: evidence from three states. Health Aff (Millwood). 33(9):1648–1654

19. Hernandez-Boussard T, Morrison D, Goldstein BA, Hsia RY (2016) Relationship of affordable care act implementation to emergency department utilization among young adults. Ann Emerg Med 67(6):714–720

20. Kozloff N, Sommers BD (2017) Insurance coverage and health outcomes in young adults with mental illness following the affordable care act dependent coverage expansion. J Clin Psychiatry 78(7):e821–e827

21. Look KA, Kim NH, Arora P (2017) Effects of the affordable care act's dependent coverage mandate on private health insurance coverage in urban and rural areas. J Rural Health 33 (1):5–11

22. McClellan S (2017) The affordable care act's dependent care coverage and mortality. Medical Care. Epub. https://doi.org/10.1097/mlr.0000000000000711

23. Miller S (2012) The effect of insurance on emergency room visits: An analysis of the 2006 Massachusetts health reform. J Public Econ 96(11):893–908

24. Mulcahy A, Harris K, Finegold K, Kellermann A, Edelman L, Sommers BD (2013) Insurance coverage of emergency care for young adults under health reform. New Engl J Med 368 (22):2105–2112

25. O'Connell JM, Towles W, Yin M, Malakar CL (2002) Patient decision making: Use of and adherence to telephone-based nurse triage recommendations. Med Decis Mak 22(4):309–317

26. O'Hara B, Brault MW (2013) The disparate impact of the ACA-dependent expansion across population subgroups. Health Serv Res 48(5):1581–1592

27. Parsons HM, Schmidt S, Tenner LL, Bang H, Keegan T (2016) Early impact of the patient protection and affordable care act on insurance among young adults with cancer: analysis of the dependent insurance provision. Cancer 122(11):1766–1773

28. Ruggles S, Alexander JT, Genadek K, Goeken R, Schroeder MB, Sobek M (2010) Integrated public use microdata series: version 5.0 [machine-readable database]. Minneapolis: University of Minnesota. https://usa.ipums.org/usa/cite.shtml

29. Saloner B, Cook BL (2014) An ACA provision increased treatment for young adults with possible mental illnesses relative to comparison group. Health Affairs (Millwood). 33(8): 1425–1434

30. Saloner B, Akosa Antwi Y, Maclean JC, Cook B (2017) Access to health insurance and utilization of substance use disorder treatment: evidence from the affordable care act dependent coverage provision. Health Econ. https://doi.org/10.1002/hec.3482

31. Scott JW, Rose JA, Tsai TC, Zogg CK, Shrime MG, Sommers BD, Salim A, Haider AH (2016) Impact of ACA insurance coverage expansion on perforated appendix rates among young adults. Med Care 54(9):818–826

32. Sommers BD, Kronick R (2012) The affordable care act and insurance coverage for young adults. J Am Med Assoc 307(9):913–914

33. Tumin D, Li SS, Kopp BT, Kirkby SE, Tobias JD, Morgan WJ, Hayes D (2017) The effect of the affordable care act dependent coverage provision on patients with cystic fibrosis. Pediatr Pulmonol 52(4):458–466

34. U.S. Census Bureau (2014) State characteristics datasets: annual estimates of the civilian population by single year of age and sex for the United States and States, 1 Apr 2010 to 1 July 2014. https://www.census.gov/popest/data/state/asrh/2014/files/SC-EST2014-AGESEX-CIV.csv

35. U.S. Department of Labor (2013) Young adults and the affordable care act: protecting young adults and eliminating burdens on business and families FAQs. http://www.dol.gov/ebsa/faqs/faq-dependentcoverage.html

36. U.S. Department of Labor (2011) Young adults and the affordable care act: protecting young adults and eliminating burdens on families and businesses. https://www.dol.gov/sites/default/files/ebsa/about-ebsa/our-activities/resource-center/fact-sheets/fsdependentcoverage.pdf

37. U.S. Department of Health and Human Services, Agency for Healthcare Research and Quality (2016) Prevention quality indicators overview. Retrieved from http://www.qualityindicators.ahrq.gov/modules/pqi_overview.aspx
38. Wallace J, Sommers BD (2015) The dependent care coverage expansion's effect on health and access to care for young adults. JAMA Pediatrics. 169(5):495–497; Aldana SG, Merrill RM, Price K et al (2005) Financial impact of a comprehensive multisite workplace health promotion program. Prev Med 40(2):131–7

The Impact of Patient Incentives on Comprehensive Diabetes Care Services and Medical Expenditures

Teresa B. Gibson, J. Ross Maclean, Ginger S. Carls, Emily D. Ehrlich, Brian J. Moore and Colin Baigel

Abstract A large nondurable goods manufacturing firm introduced a value-based insurance design health benefit program for comprehensive diabetes care with six diabetes-related service types subject to a copayment waiver: laboratory tests, physician office visits, diabetes supplies, diabetes medications, antihypertensive (blood pressure) medications, and cholesterol-lowering medications. We evaluated the impact of this natural experiment compared to a matched comparison group drawn from firms with similar composition and baseline trends. We examined the difference-in-differences impact of the program on diabetes-related services, utilization and all-cause spending. In the first year, adherence to oral diabetes medications was 15.0% higher relative to the matched comparison group ($p < 0.01$) and 14.4% higher in the second year ($p < 0.01$). The likelihood of adherence to a regimen of diabetes-related recommended diabetes care services (laboratory visits, office visits and medications) was low in the baseline year (5.8% of enrollees) and increased 92.1% in the first year ($p < 0.01$) and 82% in the second year ($p < 0.05$). The program was cost-neutral in terms of total all-cause healthcare spending (health plan plus employee out of pocket payments) and all-cause net health plan payments (both $p > 0.10$). Our analysis suggests that a comprehensive diabetes care program with patient incentives can improve care without increasing direct health plan costs.

T. B. Gibson (✉) · B. J. Moore
Truven Health Analytics, 100 Phoenix Dr., Ann Arbor, MI 48108, USA
e-mail: teresa.gibson@us.ibm.com

J. RossMaclean
Precision Health Economics, Santa Monica, CA, USA

G. S. Carls
Jazz Pharmaceuticals, San Jose, CA (Formerly of Truven Health), USA

E. D. Ehrlich
Altarum Institute, Ann Arbor, MI, USA

C. Baigel
Formerly of Bristol Myers Squibb, New York, NY, USA

© Springer International Publishing AG, part of Springer Nature 2018
P. J. Giabbanelli et al. (eds.), *Advanced Data Analytics in Health*, Smart Innovation, Systems and Technologies 93, https://doi.org/10.1007/978-3-319-77911-9_9

1   Introduction

Approximately 23.1 million persons (7.2%) in the United States have been diagnosed with diabetes, and average medical expenditures for persons with diabetes are 2.3 times higher than those without diabetes [5]. For employers, this translates into approximately $69 billion in indirect costs associated with reduced productivity [3]. In turn, prevention and management of diabetes is increasingly recognized by employers as an important strategy to improve the health of insured populations. Many companies implement such strategies through worksite wellness programs as part of their employer sponsored benefit programs, often including health risk assessment and screening [1]. In addition, these programs may include efforts to identify employees at high risk for developing diabetes, and focus on diabetes management and prevention to reduce the incidence and costs associated with the disease.

Increasingly, studies have shown value-based insurance design (VBID) programs for diabetes, benefit plan designs that typically cover evidence-based services using patient financial incentives of lowered or eliminated cost-sharing (i.e., copayments, coinsurance), are often associated with an increase in medication adherence (see review articles Lee et al. [14], Look [15] and Tang et al. [22]). To date, most research has primarily focused on evaluating the impact of programs for patients that lower cost sharing or out-of-pocket spending for prescription drugs [15, 22]. A recent review found that the largest increase in diabetes medication adherence associated with lower medication cost-sharing was 9.2%, although the largest effect reported in a controlled comparison was 8.9% [15].

Other studies have reported the impact of providing non-pharmaceutical incentives such as free test strips to patients with diabetes [13], which had little to no impact on test strip utilization. A second study analysed the impact of providing free blood glucose monitors [21], which had a positive impact on blood glucose monitoring, medication adherence and blood glucose levels. Several studies have analysed the impact of the Asheville Model [6, 8, 12], an intervention consisting of pharmacist coaching and copayment relief for diabetes medications and supplies, which reported an improvement in spending although the impact on adherence was not measured. Using an uncontrolled pre-post design Nair and colleagues [17] reported on the two-year impact of providing copayment relief for diabetes medications and test supplies and found an increase in insulin use and a decline in spending in the second year. To date no study has investigated the impact of eliminating patient cost sharing for a comprehensive regimen of recommended outpatient medical services and prescription drugs for persons with diabetes [2].

In the current study we employ a pre-post design with a matched comparison group to analyze the impact of the introduction of a comprehensive diabetes value-based benefit including six categories of incented medical and medication services with a copayment waiver ($0 patient copayment). The aim of this program was to reduce barriers to many evidence-based diabetes services [2]. The findings from this study have important implications to inform interventions aiming to improve adherence to comprehensive diabetes care.

2   Methods

In January 2011, a US nondurable goods manufacturing firm implemented an Enhanced Benefit for diabetes consisting of a copayment waiver ($0 patient copayment) for six services for individuals qualifying for the benefit: (1) diabetes medications, (2) antihypertensive (high blood pressure) medications, (3) cholesterol-lowering medications (e.g., statins), (4) diabetes-related laboratory tests (e.g., blood glucose/HbA1c), (5) office visits for diabetes care, and, (6) diabetes supplies. Prior to the enhanced benefit, cost sharing amounts for these services were: 20% coinsurance for medications, 20% coinsurance for office visits for diabetes care in the standard medical plan or $30 primary care office visit/$40 specialist visit for other plans, $30–$40 for laboratory visits (varied by plan) and 20% coinsurance for diabetes supplies.

This observational, retrospective analysis was based on a pre-post design with a matched comparison group. The experience of the intervention group and a matched comparison group of patients with diabetes were evaluated from January 2009 through December 2012, two years before and two years after program implementation.

The intervention firm data was gathered from its integrated benefits data warehouse comprised of medical insurance claims data, health plan enrolment data, prescription drug data and related data. Comparison group data was gathered from the Truven Health MarketScan Database comprised of similar integrated data contributed by over 150 large and medium-sized firms.

2.1   Comparison Group

The comparison group was selected based on two levels of matching, firm level and individual level. First, 9 firms not offering a VBID option but with similar age, gender and regional distribution of enrollees, as well as similar occupations of workers, were selected from the firms included in the Truven Health MarketScan Database, 2009–2012, as the comparison group. These firms were confirmed to have similar amounts of pre-period spending, medication adherence and utilization trends. Second, individuals in the intervention group and comparison employers were selected who had received either a diagnosis of diabetes (ICD-9-CM: 250.XX) or a prescription for an antidiabetes medication (insulin and oral hypoglycemics/antihyperglycemics) in 2010, the year prior to the intervention. All enrollees were required to have at least 18 months of continuous enrollment over the full course of the study period, 2009–2012, with at least 6 months enrollment in the post-intervention period, 2011–2012. Prior to matching, there were 444 intervention enrollees and 6,287 potential comparison enrollees.

Enrollees in the intervention group were matched 1-to-1 to enrollees in the comparison firms. Propensity scores for the probability of being in the intervention group were estimated using the predominant functional form of logistic regression

[10]. Boosting algorithm logistic regression, a decision tree-based boosting technique (a meta-classifier machine learning technique), [9, 11] was applied to propensity score estimation [16] to improve fit and eliminate the assumption of linearity in the logit allowing for higher order terms and interactions in the covariates. Propensity score models regressed a binary indicator for intervention group membership (vs. comparison group membership) on factors likely to be associated with group membership including age, gender, urban residence, employee relationship categories (employee, spouse, dependent), Charleson Comorbidity Index (CCI) [7], the number of psychiatric diagnostic groupings (PDGs) [4], 2010 adherence levels for oral diabetes, insulin, antihypertensive, and dyslipidemia medications based on the Proportion of Days Covered, 2010 direct medical expenditures, the 2009 adherence level for diabetes medications, median household income of the employee's ZIP code of residence from the American Community Survey, length and pattern of enrollment (e.g., enrolled in 2009 or 2012). We used a hybrid approach stratifying enrollees into four age group categories (18–34, 35–44, 45–54, 55–64) to ensure close matches on age. Within these age strata, enrollees were matched 1-to-1 without replacement on the estimated propensity scores, subject to a caliper of ¼ of a standard deviation in the propensity scores [20]. This resulted in 435 enrollees in both the intervention and comparison groups.

2.2   Outcome Measures

We measured adherence, utilization and spending in each calendar quarter for each enrollee. Adherence was indicated by the Proportion of Days Covered (PDC) for each medication class in the program (oral diabetes, all diabetes (oral + insulin) antihypertensive and cholesterol-lowering) indicating the percentage of days with medication on hand each quarter (from 0 to 100%), determined using fill dates and days supplied amounts on each claim [18, 19], accounting for hospitalizations and carrying over days supplied for early filling patterns. PDC is a recommended measure of adherence in many measurement programs [19]. Utilization measures included the number of fills within each medication class with all fills less than or equal to 30 days counting as 1 fill and fills with a days supplied exceeding 30 days standardized to 30 days equivalents. The number of diabetes medication supplies (non test-strip supplies) dispensed was also counted. Utilization measures also included the number of diabetes-related laboratory tests. We counted the number of physician office visits with a diabetes diagnosis code to be consistent with plan requirements of a diagnosis code of diabetes for a copayment waiver.

Spending measures included total allowed amounts (from all sources of payment including the health plan, patient and third parties) for prescription drugs and medical care. Net health plan payments were measured in total, for medical services, and prescription drugs. Out-of-pocket amounts paid by the patient for services delivered within the health plan were also measured in total, for medical services and prescription drugs. Spending amounts were based on all services delivered to patients (all cause) under the health plan.

To measure utilization of the entire regimen of enhanced benefit services, we summarized the data to annual increments for each enrollee and assessed whether each enrollee was adherent to diabetes medications (PDC $\geq$ 80%), adherent to cholesterol-lowering medications (PDC $\geq$ 80%), adherent to antihypertensive medications (PDC $\geq$ 80%) (see adherence standards in [19]), at least one diabetes-related office visit, two or more lab visits, and at least 1 fill of diabetes-related supplies (non-strip).

2.3 Estimation of Impact

To measure program impact, we estimated generalized estimating equations (GEE) [23] of the following form:

$$Y_{it} = f(a + b * Enhanced_i + c * Enhanced_i * year1_t + d * Enhanced_i * year2_t + XB_{it} + time_t)$$

where Y is each outcome measure, i is enrollee, t is time (quarter or year), Enhanced indicates the intervention firm enrollees, $year_j$ indicates the year following imple-mentation, a difference in differences framework. Covariates (XB) included gender, age groups (18–34, 35–44, 45–54, 44–64), urban area of residence, employee relationship categories, number of psychiatric diagnostic groupings and the Char-leson Comorbidity Index (both measured at baseline), and median household income in the area of residence.

GEE adherence models were estimated with a Gaussian family (i.e., assuming a normal/Gaussian distribution of the dependent variable) and an identity link function ($f = 1$), utilization models of counts were estimated with a negative binomial family/distribution and a log link ($f = exp$), and spending models were estimated with a gamma family/distribution and a log link ($f = exp$). Models account for correlation between observations using a sandwich/robust variance estimator. Regression covariates included female gender, age groups (18–34, 35–44, 45–54, 44–64), urban area of residence, employee status (vs. dependent/spouse), number of psychiatric diagnostic groupings and the Charleson Comor-bidity Index (both measured at baseline), and median household income in the ZIP code of residence from the American Community Survey, a doubly robust approach. Standard errors were adjusted for clustering by enrollee over time using an exchangeable correlation structure. We estimated the predicted value of each measure for the intervention group and comparison/counterfactual group in each year following implementation of the program. Program impact was calculated in percentage terms (the percent above or below the counterfactual).

3 Results

We found 444 enrollees in the enhanced benefit program (intervention group) and 6,287 enrollees in the comparison firms who met all selection criteria. After propensity score matching, 435 intervention enrollees (98%) were matched to enrollees in the comparison firms for a total sample size of 870. Table 1 describes

Table 1 Characteristics of intervention and matched comparison group enrollees

	Before matching			After matching		
Variables	Treatment	Comparison	p-value	Treatment	Comparison	p-value
Age 18–34	4.1%	5.9%	0.112	3.7%	3.7%	1.000
Age 35–44	14.0%	11.9%	0.189	14.0%	14.0%	1.000
Age 45–54	43.9%	30.9%	0.000	43.4%	43.4%	1.000
Age 55–64	38.1%	51.4%	0.000	38.9%	38.9%	1.000
Female	43.5%	48.4%	0.044	43.9%	48.5%	0.174
Urban residence	98.6%	92.4%	0.000	98.6%	96.8%	0.070
Enrollee relationship						
Employee	56.5%	63.3%	0.004	57.5%	58.4%	0.784
Spouse	41.4%	34.2%	0.002	40.7%	38.6%	0.533
Dependent	2.0%	2.4%	0.576	1.8%	3.0%	0.270
Charlson cormorbidity index >2	14.9%	15.0%	0.925	15.2%	14.5%	0.775
2010 medication adherence (baseline)						
Oral diabetes PDC	66.2%	72.1%	0.007	66.7%	65.7%	0.775
Insulin PDC	20.5%	21.2%	0.742	20.7%	20.2%	0.867
Antihypertensive PDC	62.2%	67.7%	0.016	63.0%	63.2%	0.944
Dyslipidemia PDC	64.6%	61.1%	0.135	65.1%	66.4%	0.669
2010 medical expenditures (baseline)	$6,482	$7,465	0.190	$5,789	$5,715	0.915
2009 diabetes adherence category						
Low: 2009 PDC < 20%	37.2%	29.3%	0.000	36.8%	34.5%	0.480
Medium: 2009 PDC = 20–79%	24.6%	22.3%	0.265	24.8%	22.1%	0.337
High: 2009 PDC ≥ 80%	35.4%	35.7%	0.882	35.4%	36.8%	0.672
Percentile of ZIP code median income from ACS						
50–75th‰	32.4%	23.1%	0.000	33.1%	24.6%	0.006
75–100th‰	52.7%	17.2%	0.000	51.7%	29.9%	0.000

Source Author's analysis of 2009–2012 intervention program data and MarketScan comparison group
Note Matching algorithms included the number of Psychiatric Diagnostic Groupings ($p = 0.038$ after matching) and enrollment patterns (e.g., enrolled in 2009, enrolled in 2012) ($p > 0.05$ after matching). Standardized Differences yielded results similar to p-values
PDC Proportion of Days Covered

the characteristics of the intervention and comparison group enrollees before and after matching. The matched groups were similar in all characteristics except the number of psychiatric diagnostic groupings and the distribution of household income ($p < 0.05$).

Pre-period trends were no different in the intervention and comparison groups ($p > 0.05$ not shown). Most of the change in cost-sharing occurred in the intervention group. Out-of-pocket payments (medical plus prescription drug) decreased 29.2% between the baseline period and the end of the second year of the program, while out of pocket payments in the comparison group increased slightly (4.17%) during the same period of time (not shown).

Based on the model estimates, in the first year after program implementation adherence to oral diabetes medications was 15% higher in the intervention group than the comparison group and 14.4% higher in the second year (both $p < 0.01$) (Table 2). Adherence to all diabetes medications, oral and insulin, was 11.9% higher in the first year and 12.2% higher in the second year (both $p < 0.01$). Adherence to antihypertensive medications and cholesterol-lowering medications were no different in the intervention and comparison groups ($p > 0.05$).

Utilization as indicated by the number of fills for oral diabetes medications was 20.2% higher in the first year in the intervention group than the comparison group and 20.7% higher in the second year ($p < 0.01$). Utilization of all diabetes medications, oral and insulin, was 19.3% higher in the first year and 18.6% higher in the second year (both $p < 0.01$). Antihypertensive medication fills were 13.6% higher in the first year in the intervention group ($p < 0.01$) than the comparison group, and were 9.4% higher in the second year ($p = 0.12$). However, fills of cholesterol-lowering medications were no different in the intervention group than the comparison group after program implementation. Fills of supplies (non-strip) were 44.8% higher in the first year ($p < 0.01$) and were 30.0% higher in the second year ($p < 0.10$).

Diabetes-related office visits were 9.7% higher in the first year in the intervention group than the comparison group ($p = 0.12$) and were 13.6% higher in the second year ($p < 0.05$). Utilization of diabetes-related laboratory tests was no different in the intervention group than the comparison group after program implementation.

The program was cost-neutral in terms of total allowed payments and total net health plan payments (prescription drug and medication payments)—payments were no different in the intervention group than in the comparison group ($p > 0.10$). Net health plan payments for prescription medications were 22.4% higher in the intervention group than the comparison group in the first year ($p < 0.01$) and 19.9% higher in the second year, although net health plan payments for medical services (inpatient and outpatient) were no different in the intervention and comparison groups.

Out-of-pocket payments were considerably lower in the intervention group than in the comparison group. For example, total all-cause out-of-pocket payments were

Table 2 Impact on adherence, utilization and spending

	Baseline	Year 1 impact (%)		Year 2 impact (%)	
Medication adherence (proportion of days covered)					
Oral diabetes	0.50	15.0	***	14.4	***
All diabetes (Oral + Insulin)	0.62	11.9	***	12.2	***
Cholesterol-lowering	0.50	−1.4		1.6	
Antihypertensive	0.51	4.3	^	2.8	
Utilization					
Number of fills per enrollee per year					
Oral diabetes	5.08	20.2	***	20.7	***
All diabetes (Oral + Insulin)	6.70	19.3	***	18.6	***
Cholesterol-lowering	3.82	1.3		8.2	
Antihypertensive	5.18	13.6	***	9.4	^
Supplies (non-test strip)	0.90	44.8	***	30.0	*
Number of diabetes-related visits or tests					
Office visits	2.48	9.7	^	13.6	*
Lab tests	7.52	3.7		10.5	
Spending per enrollee per year (all-cause)					
Total payments	$10,391	0.8		0.0	
Net payments total (Medical + Rx)	$9,401	6.0		4.6	
Net payments medical	$5,235	−4.7		−6.3	
Net payments Rx	$4,166	22.4	***	19.9	***
Out of pocket total (Medical + Rx)	$1,094	−36.5	***	−34.1	***
Out of pocket medical	$548	−22.5	***	−24.6	***
Out of pocket Rx	$546	−52.5	***	−46.9	***
Adherence to diabetes regimen of care[a] (%)	5.8	92.1	***	82.0	**

Source Author's analysis of 2009–2012 intervention program data and MarketScan comparison group

Notes $^\wedge p = 0.12$, $***p \leq 0.01$, $**0.01 < p \leq 0.05$, $*0.05 < p \leq 0.10$

a adherent to diabetes medications (PDC $\geq$ 80%), cholesterol-lowering medications (PDC $\geq$ 80%), antihypertensive medications (PDC $\geq$ 80%), at least one diabetes-related office visit, two or more lab visits, and at least 1 fill of diabetes-related supplies (non-strip)

36.5% lower in the first year, and 34.1% lower in the second year (both $p < 0.01$). Finally, after the enhanced benefit for diabetes was implemented, enrollees were 92.1% more likely to receive all of the six categories of incented services in the first year than the comparison group and 82.0% more likely in the second year (both $p < 0.01$).

4 Discussion

Diabetes care is complex and requires that many issues be addressed. A large body of evidence exists to support a multi-faceted approach to care for patients with diabetes [2]. This innovative program for diabetes care centered on copayment waivers for 6 categories of high-value diabetes services: diabetes medications, antihypertensive medications, cholesterol-lowering medications, diabetes related laboratory tests, physician office visits for diabetes care, and diabetes supplies. In the first year of the program, diabetes medication adherence was 15% higher in the intervention group than in the propensity score-matched comparison group, and 14.4% higher in the second year. These results are larger than reported in most previous studies [14, 15]. The sizable effect may be related to the unique structure of the program, which provided complimentary services such as office visits and blood glucose monitoring. In addition, applying copayment waivers to a broader array of services increases the size of the incentive to patients and the amount of incentive offered was not negligible. Previous research has found that the structure of patient incentive programs influences their ability to increase medication adherence [14, 15]. Our findings also provide additional evidence for a diabetes standard of care that includes a range of interventions to improve diabetes outcomes.

While adherence to diabetes medication increased, adherence to antihypertensive medications did not change, although the number of fills for antihypertensive medications was 13.6% higher in the first year ($p < 0.01$) and 9.4% higher than the comparison group in the second year ($p = 0.12$). Enrollees with comorbid high blood pressure and related conditions can often be prescribed more than one medication, a scenario under which the PDC is less sensitive to changes in use than the number of fills.

For cholesterol-lowering medications, while adherence and the number of fills showed no improvement, this may be explained by several factors. First, one of the more popular medications, pravastatin, had been offered to enrollees of the firm at zero copayment prior to and after the intervention. Second, another popular medication, simvastatin, was available in generic form at a low copayment during the study period, thus, the copayment waiver represented a negligible drop in price for many intervention enrollees taking cholesterol-lowering medications.

The number of diabetes-related office visits and diabetes supplies were higher after implementation, demonstrating that individual services subject to the copayment waiver also improved. Most importantly, diabetes office visits increased, indicating that the nexus of care, the face-to-face interaction between the patient and provider of care, occurred more frequently as a result of the program. The number of diabetes-related laboratory tests did not change; however, enrollees in many of the larger locations had access to free on-site medical laboratories and we did not incorporate these on-site laboratory tests into the analysis. Had the on-site visits been included, it is likely that the number of diabetes laboratory tests would have increased relative to the comparison group.

Similar to many previous studies [14] the program was cost neutral, with no change in direct health plan costs after implementation. This is important given the significant increase in utilization for high-value services. Prescription drug costs for the intervention group were 20% higher than for the comparison group in each year after the program was implemented. While medical costs did not show a statistically significant decrease to offset the increase in prescription drug costs, medical costs were lower than the comparison group, enough to result in cost neutrality of the program. In addition, intervention enrollees had considerably lower out of pocket costs for both medical care and prescription medications.

Not only did adherence and utilization rates of individual services improve, but the likelihood of receipt of all high-value services in a year showed a marked increase. This is a particularly noteworthy finding, given that diabetes management includes a broad spectrum of services including regular office visits, medication adherence, self-monitoring with diabetes supplies, and frequent laboratory tests. [2] Even though large increases were experienced for receipt of all six services, the overall rate of receipt remained very low. Future studies should investigate additional ways to increase compliance to the entire regimen of care for diabetes management, as improvements in compliance to comprehensive care are as important as improving compliance rates for individual high-value services. Future studies should also examine the relationship between copayment waivers, compliance to the regimen of care and costs, following patients over several years. These results could be used to influence how patient incentive programs are organized.

This study is not without limitations. First, we used administrative data to study program impact, where coding can be incomplete and adherence is inferred from filling patterns. In addition, calculating adherence patterns for insulin using this method can be difficult, since it is injectable and not dispensed in pill form. As such, we provide measures with and without insulin. Second, the study was performed on a single employer, which may limit the generalizability of the findings. Despite the sample size we found large and significant effects. Also, we did not have access to clinical data for enough treatment and comparison group members to analyze the clinical impact. Future work should include both clinical and patient-centered outcomes, as well employee productivity and employee engagement.

5 Conclusions

Previous studies have examined the impact of lowering copayments for diabetes medications, or in a few cases, for a few related services. We found that a copayment waiver for a diabetes regimen of care produced a large change in diabetes medication adherence. We also found that improving access to a regimen of diabetes care services by waiving copayments can improve utilization of and adherence to many high-value diabetes services—alone and in combination—without increasing health plan costs.

Acknowledgements This work was supported by Bristol-Myers Squibb. All opinions expressed are those of the authors. The study has been reviewed and approved by the New England Institutional Review Board #11-340.

Appendix: Terminology

- Copayment—Patient fee when filling a prescription or receiving a medical service
- Adherence—Compliance with a schedule of services or prescription medications
- Copayment Waiver—$0 copayment, no fee
- Cost Neutral—Generates neither a positive nor a negative effect, is neutral
- Out of Pocket—Fees paid by the patient 'out of pocket'
- (Net) Health Plan Payments—The amount paid by the health plan/insurer.

References

1. Aldana SG, Merrill RM, Price K et al (2005) Financial impact of a comprehensive multisite workplace health promotion program. Prev Med 40(2):131–137
2. American Diabetes Association (2011) Standards of care in diabetes—2011. Diabetes Care 34 (Supp 1):S11–S61
3. American Diabetes Association (2013) Economic costs of diabetes in the US in 2012. Diabetes Care 36(4):1033–1046
4. Ashcraft MLF, Fries BE, Nerenz DR et al (1989) A psychiatric patient classification system: an alternative to diagnosis-related groups. Med Care 27:543–557
5. Centers for Disease Control and Prevention (2017) National diabetes statistics report. Accessed 28 Aug 2017. https://www.cdc.gov/diabetes/pdfs/data/statistics/national-diabetes-statistics-report.pdf
6. Cranor CW, Bunting BA, Christensen DB (2003) The Asheville project: long-term clinical and economic outcomes of a community pharmacy diabetes care program. J Am Pharm Assoc 43:173–184
7. Deyo RA, Cherkin DC, Ciol MA (1992) Adapting a clinical comorbidity index for use with ICD-9-CM administrative databases. J Clin Epidemiol 45(6):613–619
8. Fera T, Bluml B, Ellis WM (2009) Diabetes ten city challenge: final economic and clinical results. J Am Pharm Assoc 46(3):e52–e60
9. Friedman J, Hastie T, Tibshirani R (2000) Additive logistic regression: a statistical view of boosting (With discussion and a rejoinder by the authors). Ann Stat 28(2):337–407
10. Guo S, Fraser MW (2010) Propensity score analysis: statistical methods and applications. SAGE Publications, Thousand Oaks, CA
11. Hastie T, Tibshirani R, Friedman J (2001) The elements of statistical learning. Springer, New York
12. Iyer R, Coderre P, McKevley T et al (2010) An employer-based, pharmacist intervention model for patients with type 2 diabetes. Am J Health Syst Pharm 67(4):312–316
13. Karter AJ, Parker MM, Moffet HH et al (2007) Effect of cost-sharing changes on self-monitoring of blood glucose. Am J Managed Care 13(7):408–416

14. Lee J, Maciejewski M, Raju S et al (2013) Value-based insurance design: quality improvement but no cost savings. Health Aff (Millwood) 32(7):1251–1257
15. Look KA (2015) Value-based insurance design and medication adherence: opportunities and challenges. Am J Managed Care 21(1):e78–e90
16. McCaffrey DF, Ridgeway D, Morral R (2004) Propensity score estimation with boosted regression for evaluating causal effects in observational studies. Psychol Methods 9(4): 403–425
17. Nair KV, Miller K, Park J et al (2010) Prescription co-pay reduction program for diabetic employees. Popul Health Manage 13(5):235–245
18. Nau D (2012) Proportion of days covered (PDC) as a preferred method of measuring medication adherence. Accessed 29 Aug 2017. http://www.pqaalliance.org/images/uploads/files/PQA%20PDC%20vs%20%20MPR.pdf
19. Pharmacy Quality Alliance (2017) Update on medication quality measures in medicare part D plan star ratings 2017. Accessed 29 Aug 2017. http://pqaalliance.org/measures/cms.asp
20. Rosenbaum PR, Rubin DB (1985) Constructing a control group using multivariate matched sampling methods that incorporate the propensity score. Am Stat 39:33–38
21. Soumerai SB, Mah C, Zhang F et al (2004) Effects of health maintenance organization coverage of self-monitoring devices on diabetes self-care and glycemic control. Arch Intern Med 164:645–652
22. Tang KL, Barneih L, Mann B et al (2014) A systematic review of value-based insurance design in chronic diseases. Am J Managed Care 20(6):e229–e241
23. Zeger SL, Liang KY, Albert PS (1988) Models for longitudinal data: a generalized estimating equation approach. Biometrics 44:1049–1060

Analyzing the Complexity of Behavioural Factors Influencing Weight in Adults

Philippe J. Giabbanelli

Abstract Managing obesity is a difficult and pressing problem given its detrimental health effects and associated healthcare costs. This difficulty stems from obesity being the result of a complex system. This complexity is often ignored by generic interventions, and not fully utilized for clinical decision-making. We focused on heterogeneity and feedback loops as key parts of this complexity. We measured heterogeneity and found it high, in a demographically homogeneous sample as well as in a larger, more varied sample. We also demonstrated that taking a systems approach could hold value for clinical decision-making. Specifically, we showed that feedback loops had better associations with weight categories than individual factors or relationships, in addition to clear implications for weight dynamics. Clinical implications were discussed, in part through adapting techniques such as card decks in a computerized format. Further research was suggested on heterogeneity among population groups and categories of driver of weight.

1 Introduction

Obesity is a major public health issue in Canada, with associated healthcare costs in billions of dollars [1] and still growing [2]. As obesity is a chronic disease, finding long-term solutions is critical. However, current interventions have found that individuals struggle to maintain successful weight loss beyond the first few years [3]. For example, a review of multicomponent behavioural weight management programmes (i.e., including diet, physical activity, and behavioural therapy) found a mean loss of 2.59 kg after 12 months (between intervention and control groups) but this loss was already reduced to 1.54 at 18 or 24 months [4]. This difficulty comes from the fact that obesity is the result of a complex system [5–7]. This system can be approached in several ways, from population-level perspectives such as the Foresight Obesity Map [8] to individual-centric perspectives [9]. In addition, given that the causes and consequences of obesity are extremely broad, system maps may include themes such

P. J. Giabbanelli (✉)
Computer Science Department, Furman University, Greenville, SC 29613, USA
e-mail: giabbanelli@gmail.com

© Springer International Publishing AG, part of Springer Nature 2018
P. J. Giabbanelli et al. (eds.), *Advanced Data Analytics in Health*, Smart Innovation,
Systems and Technologies 93, https://doi.org/10.1007/978-3-319-77911-9_10

as food production and consumption, physiology (e.g., functioning of the adipose tissue) or psychology (e.g., weight stigma, emotional eating).

In this chapter, we take an individual-centric perspective to understand the many behavioural factors that are part of the system shaping obesity in individuals. Many features contribute to making this system complex. First, we face the presence of numerous *feedback loops*: acting on one factor will propagate through other factors and ultimately return to the initial factor to produce another change. Such loops have been abundantly illustrated in the case of obesity [8, 9]. For example, several loops work through stigmatization, which is very prevalent for obesity [10]. As obese individuals are stigmatized, they may experience negative emotions, for which coping mechanisms may include eating and further weight gain. Similarly, workplace discrimination [11] causes wage penalty for obese employees (e.g., by being paid less than non-obese employees for the same position) which contributes to a lower socioeconomic position, which itself can affect obesity. Loops contribute to the difficulty of managing obesity, by opposition to simpler systems made of causal chains.

A second important hallmark of complexity is the presence of *heterogeneity*, that is, the tremendous variations found among people. As small differences in personality and context can lead to widely diverging outcomes [12], heterogeneity contributes to the difficulty of creating efficient healthy-weight interventions. While there are other contributors to the complexity of obesity [5] such as non-linearity, this chapter is primarily concerned with the presence of heterogeneity and feedback loops. Body weight is shaped by a multitude of psychological, social and biological factors [8, 13] whose interaction create numerous loops, and whose many combinations of values result in a large heterogeneity.

The complexity of obesity has been over-simplified by 'one size fits all' interventions which assume an average individual profile and simplify the multitude of interacting drivers of weight as a mere matter of trying to "eat less and exercise more" [14–16]. Practitioners have observed that, in such generic treatments, success only occurs at random through the chance of correctly matching a patient to an intervention [17, 18]. This is reflected in a paradigm shift from generic treatments assuming homogeneity (i.e., an average profile) to very comprehensive treatments that seek to capture the heterogeneity of patients by integrating their values, experiences and perspectives [19]. This comprehensive approach can be seen in the 5 As of Obesity Management™ of the Canadian Obesity Network. At the same time, several tools have been proposed to empower people in the management of their well-being by describing the system in which they live. This is exemplified by *Life Game* developed by Mindbloom™ and reviewed in [20, 21].

These new approaches provide ways to capture heterogeneity and to understand the interactions between the drivers of weights. However, they may not be straightforward to employ with patients. Practitioners have emphasized that extracting and analyzing each individual's system could be an overwhelming task, taking a considerable amount of time and having to navigate a 'maze' of factors [22]. While automatic procedures have been proposed to assist with that exercise [20], supporting their widespread use would be a significant effort. Therefore, we face a simple question: do we really need to capture heterogeneity and each patient's system? This is an important research question as it asks about the value of taking a systems science approach in obesity research. The consequences of the answer can suggest very different approaches: while a "no" would mean that the same approach can be applied to all individuals, a "yes" would point to the need to segment interventions and allocate more resources to understanding the specificities of each patient. To find where the answer lies, this chapter assesses the extent to which individuals are heterogeneous, and examines whether there is value for clinical decision-making in knowing a patient's system. Our focus is on the system centered on the patient's behaviours (i.e., food behaviours and physical activity behaviours). This system can be obtained during treatment in the clinical setting through self-reports during a consultation or forms filled prior to an appointment. It could also be obtained independently using tools focused on well-being and available to all, such as *Life Game* developed by Mindbloom™. For other systems governing weight, such as physiological components, we refer the reader to [23, 24].

> The main contributions of this chapter are twofold:
>
> - We explain the theoretical motivation for taking a systems approach to obesity, demonstrate how to perform it in detail (including the design of questionnaires and recruitment of participants), and analyze the significance of results for clinical decision-making.
> - Our work can be used to guide the development of conceptual models for obesity, which may be extended as either simulation models or computerized tools to assist with weight management in a clinical setting.

In the Materials and Methods section, we explain how we operationalize heterogeneity and how we structured the behavioural system. We also detail how two groups of participants were recruited, and provide their characteristics. In the Results section, we report on the heterogeneity of both groups and on information gained by analyzing feedback loops. Then, we discuss these results in light of implications for the management of obesity from a systems perspective. Finally, we conclude by summarizing our contributions and potential avenues for future work.

2 Materials and Methods

2.1 Estimation of Heterogeneity

In this study, individuals provide self-assessed measures of factors related to their weight. For each factor, we thus need to measure the extent to which individuals differ in their answers. There are numerous measures for this task, which is reflected in a variety of diversity, richness, and evenness indices. While some measures can be simply defined, their interpretation may not be as straightforward. For example, imagine that we measure how often individuals' self-reported factors differ from one another. If a factor was measured using two values (e.g., endorsed/not endorsed) then, in a totally different population, there would be a 50% chance that answers differ. If instead the factor was measured through five values (e.g., disagree, slightly disagree, neither agree nor disagree, slightly agree, agree), then answers may differ 80% of the time (as there is $100/5 = 20\%$ chance for each answer). Consequently, the interpretation of such simple measures may heavily depend on the design of the questionnaire. This can be problematic for measures such as unalikeability [22], which has been used in a pilot study on heterogeneity [23]. Therefore, we will use a measure that can be straightforwardly interpreted to know how close people's answers are for each question.

Consider a question X where the possible answers $x_1, \ldots, x_n$ are taken with probabilities $p(x_1), \ldots, p(x_n)$ by the respondents. Shannon Entropy (also known as Shannon Diversity Index) is defined as:

$$H(X) = - \sum_{i=1}^{n} p(x_i) \times log_2 p(x_i) \tag{1}$$

where $0 \times log_2 0$ is taken to be 0.

Shannon's equitability index (also named Pielou's evenness index) is defined as:

$$E(X) = \frac{H(X)}{log_2 n} \tag{2}$$

The equitability index takes values between 0 and 1 where 1 means that all choices to the question were equally endorsed, and 0 means that everyone had the same answer. Therefore, we interpret larger values as revealing more heterogeneity.

2.2 Factors Contributing to Obesity from a Systems Perspective

When taking a systems approach to understanding what drives one's weight, we seek to articulate a set of causal relationships. For example, this would tell us that when the individual experiences body shape concerns, it causes stress; and that a coping mechanism for stress is to eat. Articulating these relationships is similar to creating a causal loop diagram in system dynamics: it tells us about the broad functioning of the system. However, questionnaires do not typically take this system perspective by assessing causal relationships. Instead, they more often assess individual factors. For example, they would ask whether an individual is stressed, but not what contributed to or may result from the stress. Part of the avoidance of "because" questions owes to the assumption that individuals cannot accurately assess the causes of their behaviours. This assumption is found in theories that emphasize the role of unconscious thoughts, ranging from the work of Freud in the 19th century [24] to research undertook by Nisbett and Wilson in the late 70s [25]. However, the recent decades have seen a growing amount of psychological systems in which individuals can reach a clear understanding of the mechanisms driving some of their actions [26]. This has been increasingly popular in the recent years as part of the 'mental models' created during participatory modeling processes [27–30]. The ability for individuals to clearly understand the mechanisms was also confirmed by empirical evidence in which individuals carefully depicted the influence of different factors based on complex internal schematics [31]. Furthermore, the idea that individuals can connect causes and consequences of behaviours has been adopted in obesity research both in Canada and the UK. For example, decks of cards were created and included causal mechanisms that individuals could pick to state that they were important for them [32, 33]. In addition, the field of computational modelling has emphasized that models of complex social phenomena should be built using all evidence available, which includes participants' generated-evidence about causes of their behaviour [34]. Therefore, our work included an assessment of both relationships and individual factors, with an emphasis on the relationships to achieve a systems perspective. The full survey can be accessed at http://websurvey.sfu.ca/survey/142092729.

The individual factors are personality traits, which were found to be strongly associated with weight in a longitudinal study spanning over 50 years [35]. For example, it included questions on impulsiveness such as "act on impulse", "get overwhelmed by emotions", "make plans and stick to them", "feel things are out of my control". Each of the 12 questions presents participants with a statement, and asks them to select how accurately it describes them using a 5-point scale.

Relationships were evaluated by asking individuals to evaluate how each relationship applies to them via a 5-point scale. A total of 42 relationships were reviewed; they are summarized and categorized in Fig. 1 where '+' and '−' indicate that individuals were asked whether the presence of a factor respectively increases or decreases another factor. For example, individuals were asked whether being with "friends who eat a lot" causes them to eat more. Note that in several cases, the same input factor could both be involved in an increase or a decrease of one target factor. For example, individuals were asked whether feeling lethargic causes them to eat more, and also whether feeling lethargic causes them to eat less. This is motivated by the evidence that the same input can lead to widely diverging outcomes for individuals, e.g. a wide body of evidence has shown that the presence of stress could be involved in eating more as well as in eating less [9]. The relationships surveyed cover several domains of weight, such as individual psychology, social environment, socio-economic position and education. For each domain, questions were adapted from previously validated questionnaires that took a comprehensive approach. Questions related to eating were adapted from the Yale Food Addiction Scale [36], the Binge Eating Scale,[1] the Three-Factor Eating Questionnaire [37] and recently tested

---

[1]http://psychology-tools.com/binge-eating-scale/.

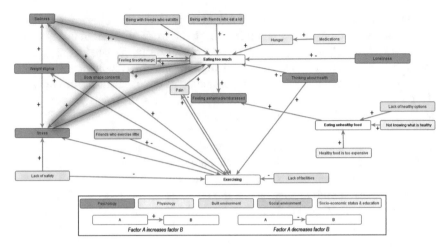

Fig. 1 System participating to obesity and assessed for each participant. Feedback loops are highlighted in red

questionnaires [32]. Questions relevant to exercising were adapted from the Exercise Motivations Inventory[2] and the Multidimensional Outcome Expectations for Exercise Scale [38].

Note that there is a variety of models that took a systems thinking approach to synthesize the factors and relationships at work in obesity. These models emphasized different aspects, thus they would generate different questions if they were used in place of the model depicted in Fig. 1. The Foresight Obesity Map [8] served as a tool for decision-making across policymakers in the UK, thus it had many factors and relationships on food production and consumption. While these certainly impact what individuals ultimately eat, these factors are very distal and difficult for individuals to reflect on, leading us to focus on more proximal factors from well-established questionnaires. Our model is closer to the ones developed in [6, 39, 40], which emphasized social norms and well-being in the context of obesity. Several other models are listed in [41] with an emphasis on food behaviours, while [42, 43] provide examples of (system dynamics) models with a focus on the physiological dynamics of weight change.

2.3 Recruitment and Characteristics of Participants

We recruited two samples of participants: a small sample where individuals are expected to be demographically similar, and a larger sample with more diversity. Ethics approval was obtained to recruit both samples. Their demographic distribu-

---

[2]http://www.livingstrong.org/articles/ExerciseMotivations.pdf.

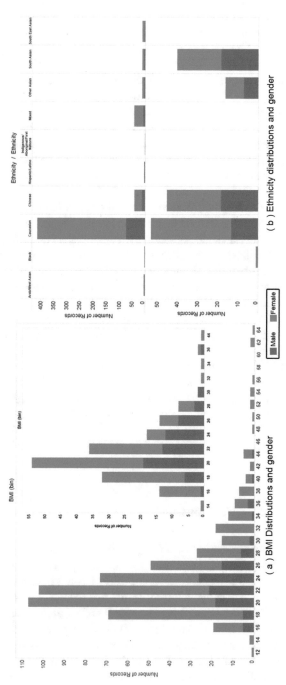

Fig. 2 The larger sample (n = 538) has more varied demographics than the smaller sample (n = 187) as illustrated by the BMI distribution (**a** smaller sample as inset) or ethnicity distribution (**b** smaller sample at the bottom). BMI histograms are coherent with other reported distributions showing a significant right skew in Canadian adults [46]. As online venues focused on weight management were part of our recruitment strategy, we observe that the long-tail of our distribution going up to a BMI of 64 is also in line with baseline data from studies on weight-loss programs such as the ongoing WRAP trial [47]

tions are summarized in Fig. 2. The small sample was recruited from September to November 2012. These were all students at Simon Fraser University, Canada, either taking a kinesiology course or majoring in kinesiology. Students were invited to participate by their course instructors. Participation was not mandatory, and no monetary compensation was offered. Three versions of the questionnaire were tested with different phrasing. In our result, we will focus on the version where answers were chosen as frequency (i.e., never, rarely, sometimes, very often, always), as this is the same questionnaire that was administered to the larger sample. A total of 187 participants (aged 17–28; mean 19.96 ± 1.91) completed the study, of whom 67 completed the frequency questionnaire. The other questionnaires and the impact of question phrasing is part of the Discussion section, and the heterogeneity with the other questionnaires is also provided in the Results section for comparison.

A larger sample of Canadian adults was recruited online from November 2013 to January 2014. No monetary compensation was offered. A total of 538 participants (aged 19–76; mean 33.26 ± 13.39) completed the study. This cohort does not aim to be representative of the Canadian population: for example, it is significantly younger than the average Canadian [44], which may be due to process of online data collection and advertising the study through online channels. Similarly, our sample had a much higher prevalence of chronic conditions than the general population, as 67% of our participants reported having at least 1 chronic condition while this occurs for 33% in the general Canadian population [45]. Consequently, even greater heterogeneity is to be expected in the general population. Given that the "vast majority of people with chronic conditions have a regular medical doctor and visit community-based doctors and nurses frequently" [45], most of our sample would be expected to receive regular medical care. However, our data is not sufficient to accurately infer the specific resources that participants may have ultimately used, such as weight management programs.

3   Results

3.1   Assessment of Heterogeneity

Heterogeneity is summarized in Fig. 3 for the different samples and types of questions. Overall, heterogeneity is large: the vast majority (43 of 54 questions) have a heterogeneity of over 0.7 (vertical black line), where larger values mean that the different answers are more equally endorsed. While heterogeneity was lower than 0.7 for a single personality questions, it was lower for 9 of the questions assessing causal relationships. Intuitively, this indicates that individuals may be very different in who they are, but not as much in how they work. Furthermore, even when individuals are expected to be more similar (e.g., students at the same location, studying the same topics, and within a close age range), a large heterogeneity remains (Fig. 3; orange squares).

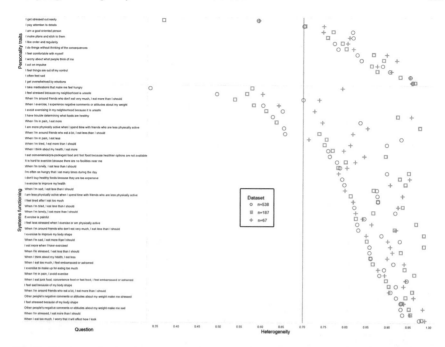

Fig. 3 Heterogeneity for all questions and all samples: a small sample with homogeneous demographics (n = 187) which was given asked the questions using three different phrasings (including one assessing for frequency, n = 67), and a larger sample with more varied demographics (n = 538). Within each type (systems functioning, personality traits), questions are sorted from least to most heterogeneous; the display is thus not indicative of any convergence

We investigated whether heterogeneity was different based on ethnic groups or educational attainments (as a proxy for socio-economic position) in the larger data set. This served to test whether heterogeneity could be reduced by targeting more demographically homogeneous groups. Three ethnic groups were retained for the analysis (Caucasian, n = 412; Chinese; n = 40, Mixed; n = 42) as all other groups had only 10 participants or less (Fig. 2b-top). Results confirm that a large heterogeneity remains even when looking at ethnically homogeneous groups (Fig. 4). Factors for which the heterogeneity was less than 0.7 in a given ethnic groups also all had a heterogeneity less than 0.7 for the overall survey groups (Fig. 3). In other words, ethnically homogeneous groupings do not strongly affect heterogeneity.

For socio-economic position, Galobardes et al. posit that there is no best indicator suitable for all study aims [48]. That is, the proxy for socio-economic position needs to be informed for example by the life course. As the mean age of our participants was 33.26, we used *educational attainments* which are considered a valid indicator for young adulthood and also strongly determine future employment and income (which serve as proxy for the socio-economic position during the active professional life phase) [48]. Educational attainments are also frequently used in epidemiology, thus facilitating comparison across studies. For educational attainments, we retained

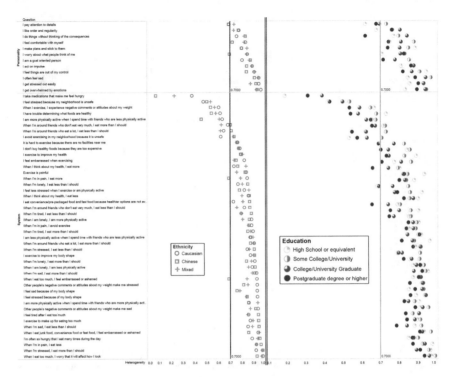

Fig. 4 Heterogeneity in the larger survey (n = 538) for the three main ethnic groups and four main categories of educational achievements (used as proxy for socio-economic position)

4 groups (high school or equivalent, n = 29; some college/university, n = 198; college/university graduate, n = 162; postgraduate degree or higher, n = 146). The fifth group or vocational/technical school was not retained due to having less than 10 participants. Educational attainments were able to create more homogeneous groups than ethnicity. We also observed a dose-response effect on systems relationships where knowledge was important: for example, the higher the educational attainment and the less the heterogeneity to "I have trouble determining what foods are healthy" (given that participants are increasingly able to identify healthy foods). We also note that the group with highest educational attainments often had the lowest heterogeneity. This group could be presenting itself in a more positive light due to a differential social desirability bias by socio-economic position, which would further limit the impact of educational attainments on heterogeneity.

3.2　Value of Knowing an Individual's System

In this chapter, the feedback loops that we studied were related to emotional eating. That is, eating in response to emotional cues, such as negative emotions [49]. Emotional eating is associated with weight gain [50] and is considered fairly common [51], thus serving as a good example for loops. The two feedback loops studied involved emotional eating either through sadness or stress. In the first loop, overeating was hypothesized to create concerns about body shape, which could translate to feelings of sadness, for which a coping mechanism is eating. Similarly, in the second loop, over-eating also created concerns about body shape, but these led to stress, for which the coping mechanism was also eating. We examined how each of the three relationships in the loop related to participants' weight status compared to the loop as a whole. The value of the loop as a whole was derived from the data by summing the values of the three relationships on a scale from 0 ("never") to 1 ("always"). For example, a participant who answered "never" (0) to the relationship eating → concerns about body shape, "never" (0) to the relationship body shape → sadness, and "always" (1) to the relationship sadness → eating, would have a total score of $0 + 0 + 1 = 1$ for the feedback loop on emotional eating through sadness.

North American healthcare professionals tend not to provide weight loss advice on patients who are not yet obese [52], and only 42% of obese patients reported being advised to lose weight over one year [53]. Consequently, our examination focused on patients who reported having at least one chronic condition, as this is more likely to trigger discussions about weight management in a clinical setting. Results are summarized in Fig. 5 for the loop on emotional eating through sadness. For the overall loop (Fig. 5d), an increasing score is associated with strictly decreasing proportions of underweight and normal weight individuals. These two categories are ruled out for a maximum score (3), while the underweight category is ruled out at a score of 2.25. This indicates that this loop is very relevant to overweight and obese patients. Given that it is a reinforcing loop, detecting its presence and addressing it through appropriate counseling would be an important goal in patients. Looking at any one relationship included in the loop was less informative given that its impact on the patient's weight depend on the presence of the two other relationships. Indeed, as each relationship was increasingly endorsed, the proportions of underweight and normal weight individuals were not strictly decreasing (Fig. 5a–c), and a large amount of such individuals could still be found for strongly endorsed relationships. Similar patterns were found in the relationship centered on stress.

In addition to comparing how informative loops were versus their individual relationships, we examine the value of individual factors related to these relationships (Fig. 6). These individual factors do not exhibit clear patterns with respect to weight status, while relationships expressed such patterns. Implications for clinicians, and in particular the possibility of extracting loops without resorting to administering and analyzing a battery of tests, are provided in the discussion.

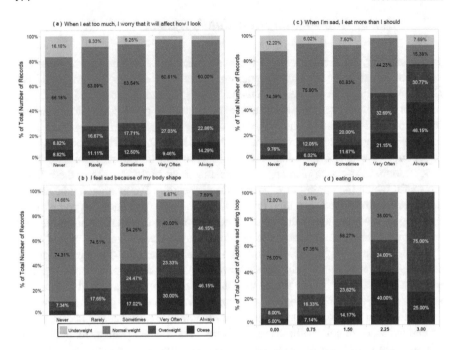

Fig. 5 Weight status based on answers for patients with at least one chronic condition. Figures a-c show the answer for each part of a feedback loop: eating impacting concerns about body shape (**a**), body shape concerns causing sadness (**b**), and sadness causing further eating (**c**). An aggregate measure for the feedback loop as a whole is provided in (**d**)

3.3 Potential Confounders

We assessed whether the answers to the questions depended on the question's phrasing. In the smaller dataset (n = 187), participants were randomly assigned to one of three versions of the survey. These versions assessed relationships by asking participants (i) how much they endorsed each relationship (n = 56), (ii) how *frequently* each relationship applied (n = 67), (iii) how *strong* each relationship was (n = 64). For example, the relationship from eating too much to feeling tired/lethargic had the three following versions:

(i) I feel lethargic/tired as a result of eating too much. [never like me—always like me]

(ii) How often do you feel lethargic/tired as a result of eating too much? [never—always]

(iii) After I eat too much, I feel [not at all lethargic/tired—extremely lethargic/tired].

Effect of phrasing on participants' responses was analysed using JMP 10.0.0 SAS Insititute Inc. Chi square was calculated for each question to compare the distribution of responses for each variation of phrasing. For contingency tables where the

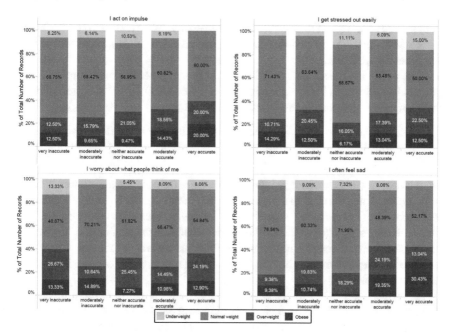

Fig. 6 Weight status based on answers for patients with at least one chronic condition, for four individual factors (impulsivity, self-conscious, stress, sadness)

expected value was <5, Fisher's Exact test was used in place of chi square. There was strong evidence ($p < 0.05$, DF = 8) of a difference in the distribution of participants' responses. Questions phrased in terms of strength yielded less answers, and the answers that were provided were often the most different compared to frequency or endorsement. Consequently, the larger dataset phrased questions in terms of frequency.

4   Discussion

4.1   Value of a Systems Approach

Obesity has been recognized as a complex problem in part because of heterogeneity and the presence of feedback loops [5]. Practitioners have long pointed out the need to better understand and account for what they perceived as the tremendous heterogeneity of their patients [17, 18]. Our work contributes to this understanding by measuring heterogeneity. We found a high degree of heterogeneity regarding perception of factors related to body weight in a sample relatively homogeneous in age and education as well as in a larger, more demographically diverse, sample. Ethnically homogenous groups had little effect on heterogeneity, while educational attainments were able to create groups whose heterogeneity was often still large but reduced from the general population.

This work also contributes to debates over the presence of heterogeneity and its potential implications for weight management. Several authors have proposed that individuals are quite similar and that general changes should be emphasized:

> It makes little sense to expect individuals to behave differently than their peers; it is more appropriate to seek a general change in behavioural norms and in the circumstances which facilitate their adoption. [54]

On the contrary, our results highlight that there *are* tremendous differences between individuals. This confirms the hypothesis that "there are likely to be considerable variations in the explanatory models held" by individuals about their weight [55]. Our work thus adds to the evidence that there should be a range of options for weight-management. Consequently, interventions aiming at making a "general change" can be a useful complement but they cannot be the sole focus in the over-arching aim of addressing obesity.

As software are increasingly being offered and proposed to capture the system that drives one's condition, such as overweight and obesity [7, 20, 21, 26], we also questioned how informative such a system would be. In other words, does a systems approach to the behavioural factors influencing weight provide additional information of interest for clinical decision-making and patient treatments? We found that reinforcing feedback loops were clearly patterned in terms of weight status. That is, as patients increasingly expressed these loops, they were also increasingly likely to be overweight or obese and less likely to be of normal weight or underweight. Given that the presence of such loops is associated with weight, and that from a systems viewpoint these reinforcing loops cause further weight gain, knowing whether patients express them is of high interest for treatment. Knowing whether patients had some of the individual relationships that composed the loops was less valuable as knowing whether a relationship is a causal driver of weight gain depends on the other relationships of the loops. This was confirmed by the patterns of weight status as a function of individual relationships, where underweight and normal weight categories were not strictly decreasing as relationships were increasingly endorsed, and/or were still found when participants strongly endorsed relationships that may cause weight gain. A similar investigation was performed by comparing patterns of weight depending on individual factors with patterns based on relationships. We found the relationships (i.e. the causal edges) to be more clearly associated with health outcomes than either of their endpoints (i.e. individual factors).

These results support the idea that a systems perspective is valuable to understand and thus better address some of the behavioural drivers of weight. The quality of information increases as we go higher in the system, from individual factors to feedback loops. This suggests that capturing each individual's system and analyzing it could contribute to the process of clinical decision-making.

4.2 Consequences for Clinical Decision-Making

Taking a systems approach with an emphasis on loops has practical consequences for weight management, both when assessing a patient and when designing a treatment. In addition, the consequences depend on the health system and type of practitioner. This section starts by discussing the consequences on assessment, first for clinical psychologists and then for primary care doctors. We conclude on how changes in assessment should be mirrored by changes in treatment.

Clinical psychologists and other mental health professionals already assess patients' behaviours as it relates to obesity, through an array of cognitive and behavioural therapies that provide effective conduits for behaviour change. In their review of clinical and health psychologists in the United States, Bean and colleagues noted this assessment needs to take into account cultural, psychological as well as physiological factors associated with obesity [56]. Given the wide array of factors under consideration, emphasizing loops over their individual components may help clinical psychologists in navigating the large and complex system of obesity.

Emphasizing loops would also be beneficial for primary care doctors, but for different reasons than for clinical psychologists. Primary care doctors are placed at the front lines in addressing the obesity problem, but they may have received limited training in obesity [57] which in turn can limit their ability to understand the many pathways that contribute to obesity [15]. It has been noted that reducing the gap between a practitioner's conceptualization of obesity and that of patients' is highly beneficial in addressing the patients' essential needs [58, 59]. Providing practitioners with selected and well-understood loops could thus serve as a focused means to bridging the gap.

Taking a systems approach in understanding the problem should be mirrored by a systems approach when designing solutions. For example, finding the specific loops that contribute to one's weight gain would be of little use if the solution was then the generic "eat less and move more". Similarly, finding loops but coming back to individual traits at the solution stage would not fully adopt a systems approach. Consequently, the solution should include managing the loops found at the assessment stage. This management can take several forms, from trying to break the loops by looking at its individual components, to encouraging competing loops or changing the type of loops (e.g., from amplifying to balancing). However, managing loops in the context of obesity is a notoriously difficult problem. It was suggested that "new methods are likely required to assist stakeholders in [...] creating new feedback loops as a means to shifting the dominance away from [the loops that] currently give rise to obesity" [5]. Thus, adopting a systems approach when performing an assessment may be the easiest part, with readily available methods, but best translating it into solutions for patients calls for the development of innovative decision-support systems.

4.3   The Need for Automation

Currently tested approaches to weight management in a clinical setting include card-sorting techniques. These consist of presenting participants with a deck of cards, where each card provides a statement. Cards are then sorted in order to establish what matters most to the participant. While cards have provided a mixture of relationships (e.g. in [32], "I often eat too much and feel uncomfortable", "When I see, smell, or have a small taste of food, I find it very difficult to keep from eating") and individual factors, the previous section suggests that examining loops could be of particular interest. However, physical card decks don't allow for an immediate extraction of feedback loops. This could be addressed through computerized approaches in which statements are selected through a software. That is, after having selecting all 'virtual' cards, the software could immediately provide a summary of the individuals factors, relationships and loops. This could also be combined with techniques such as recommender systems which simplify the process of finding statements relevant to a patient [20].

A range of other clinical approaches to weight management could benefit from such computerized and systems approaches. Approaches that operate within a multiple-causality framework could benefit from automatically extracting loops. For example, the *problem-solving model* acknowledges that there are many variables causally involved in obesity, and it advocates for a general-systems approach in which relationships are assessed rather than variables in isolation [60]. Knowing where loops lie could contribute to understanding, and eventually addressing, the circumstances that may have resulted in weight gain. Individualized approaches that work on a one-on-one basis with participants to identify behavioural and cognitive barriers to weight loss, such as Module III in the *Cognitive-Behavioural Therapy* [61], would similarly benefit from an approach that adaptively guides participants in finding relevant problems rather than using the same checklist for all.

In summary, there is currently a paucity of computerized approaches that bring a systems thinking approach to the personalized management of overweight and obesity. Some software take a systems thinking approach, whether implicitly or explicitly, such as *Life Game* from Mindbloom^{TM} or ActionableSystems (described in another chapter). However, they are not specialized to assist with the management of overweight and obesity, and they do not entirely match the target audience of this chapter. For instance, *Life Game* is designed for individuals, but not for patients and practitioners. ActionableSystems targets policymakers, and not for individuals from the general population. Most recently, we developed a software that assists patients in identifying the relationships related to weight dynamics [26], but the results were meant for a clinical trial rather than for a personalized treatment. The potential for computerized approaches is clear: it can save time and resources while providing additional systems insight. However, fulfilling this potential remains an ongoing research goal.

4.4 Limitations and Further Investigation

Our results do not aim to generalize to the Canadian population, as they were obtained through online surveys and advertised in part on venues related to weight management. Consequently, a larger study of a nationally representative sample would be needed to confirm heterogeneity in the Canadian population. A larger sample could also complement our analysis in terms of the impact of ethnicity on heterogeneity, as only three groups were sufficiently large in our sample. We also found that 'answers' were affected by the way in which questions were asked. Asking questions in terms of strength (e.g., "after I eat too much, I feel [not at all lethargic/tired extremely lethargic/tired]") was found to produce answers much different than the other two phrasings, and also resulted in more missing answers. Consequently, the main sample for this study was provided questions in terms of frequency rather than strength. It is thus possible that future studies using alternative phrasing could find different answers, although we expect the main findings of high heterogeneity and usefulness in a system perspective to remain.

Further investigation could assess other feedback loops and examine which themes trigger the most heterogeneity (e.g., body image, peer influences). This would be conducted through more extensive questionnaires, which would allow to elaborate on the relationships measured here. Comparing heterogeneity across themes has practical consequences: if a policy focuses on one theme and finds that participants tend to be homogeneous, then a generic intervention might still have value. Similarly, future research should examine what are the population groups with the most homogeneous answers. Techniques have recently been developed to obtain the expected behavioural response to an intervention based on 'questionnaires' [26], and they could be used to search for homogeneous groups. Finally, given the heterogeneity found among participants, there is always the risk that relationships that are particularly important to a few patients are not captured in decision-making systems. It would thus be of particular interest to give participants the option to also provide open-ended answers, and to then extract new relationships using text analytics. While some techniques are currently available to do this [62], their accuracy may still have to improve until they are incorporated as part of tools for clinical decision-making.

5 Conclusions

We designed and analysed surveys on behavioural drivers of weight from a systems perspective. We found that a systems perspective could provide valuable information for clinical decision-making, with better information gained by going up in the system, from individual drivers of weight to loops. We also found high heterogeneity among participants, which supports the move away from generic treatments into highly segmented interventions. Further research was suggested to assess heterogeneity across population groups and themes, and practical tools were proposed for a clinical setting.

Acknowledgements The author is indebted to Prof. Diane T. Finegood, who pioneered research in systems thinking and obesity, and inspired this line of work. The data analysis presented here was made possible by the significant effort of many instructors at Simon Fraser University in recruiting participants: Anne-Kristina Arnold, Craig Asmundson, Diana Bedoya, Penelope Deck, Leah Esplen, Tony Leyland, Mike Walsh, and Matt White. Finally, the author thanks Amy Child at the University of Cambridge for extensive feedback on this manuscript, as well as Jean Adams and James Woodcock for suggestions.

References

1. Anis A, Zhang W, Bansback N, Guh D, Amarsi Z, Birmingham C (2010) Obes Rev 11(1):31
2. Katzmarwyk P, Janssen I (2014) Can J Appl Physiol Rev Can de Physiol Appl 29(1):90
3. C.I. for Health information (2011)
4. Hartmann-Boyce J, Johns D, Aveyard P, Onakpoya I, Jebbs S, Phillips D, Ogden J, Summerbell C (2013) Managing overweight and obesity in adults lifestyle management services. NICE Guidelines PH53
5. Finegood D (2011) The Oxford handbook of the social science of obesity, pp 208–236
6. Verigin T, Giabbanelli PJ, Davidsen PI (2016) In: Proceedings of the 49th annual simulation symposium (Society for computer simulation international, 2016), ANSS'16, pp 9:1–9:10
7. Giabbanelli P, Flarsheim R, Vesuvala C, Drasic L (2016) Obes Rev 17:194
8. Vandenbroeck I, Goossens J, Clemens M (2007) Government Office for Science, UK Governments Foresight Programme
9. Giabbanelli PJ, Tornsney-Weir T, Mago VK (2012) Appl Soft Syst 12:3711
10. Puhl R, Heuer C (2009) Obesity 17(5):941
11. Puhl R, Brownell K (2001) Obes Res 9(12):788
12. Resnicow K, Vaughan R (2006) Int J Behav Nutr Phys Act 3(25)
13. Giabbanelli P, Torsney-Weir T, Finegood D (2011) Can J Diabetes 35(2):201
14. Davis R, Turner L (2001) J Am Acad Nurse Pract 13(1):15
15. Low A, Bouldin M, Sumrall C, Loustalot F, Land K (2006) Am J Med Sci 331(4):175
16. Shiffman S, Sweeney C, Pillitteri J, Sembower M, Harkins A, Wadden T (2009) Prev Med 49:482
17. Epstein L, Myers M, Raynor H, Saelens B (1998) Pediatrics 101(2):554
18. Harkaway J (2000) Fam Syst Health 18(1):55
19. Carman K, Dardess P, Maurer M, Sofaer S, Adams K, Bechtel C, Sweeney J (2013) Health Aff 32(2):223
20. Giabbanelli PJ, Crutzen R (2015) Health Inf J 21(3):223
21. Giabbanelli PJ, Deck P, Andres L, Schiphorst T, Finegood DT (2013) In: Digital human modeling and applications in health, safety, ergonomics, and risk management. Healthcare and safety of the environment and transport. Springer, pp 189–196
22. Kader G, Perry M (2007) J Stat Edu 15(2)
23. Deck P, Giabbanelli P, Finegood DT (2013) Can J Diabetes 37:S269
24. Gross R (2012) Psychology: the science of mind and behaviour. Hodder Education
25. Nisbett R, Wilson T (1977) Psychol Rev 84(3):231
26. Giabbanelli PJ, Crutzen R (2014) BMC Med Res Methodol 14(1):130
27. Gray S, Gray S, Kok JLD, Helfgott AE, O'Dwyer B, Jordan R, Nyaki A (2015) Ecol Soc 20(2):11
28. Gray S, Chan A, Clark D, Jordan R (2012) Ecol Model 229:88

29. Nyaki A et al (2014) Conserv Biol 28(5):1403
30. Jordan R, Gray S, Sorensen A, Pasewark S, Sinha S, Hmelo-Silver C (2017) Front ICT 4(7) (2017)
31. Parrott R, Silk K, Condit C (2003) Soc Sci Med 53:1099
32. Merth T, Matteson C, Finegood D (2011) Can J Diabetes 35(2)
33. Pennington J (2006) J Diabetes Nurs 10(7):261
34. Edmonds B, Moss S (2005) Lect Notes Comput Sci 3415:130
35. Sutin A, Ferrucci L, Zonderman A, Terracciano A (2011) J Personal Soc Psychol 101(3):579
36. Gearhardt A, White A, Masheb R, Morgan P, Crosby R, Grilo C (2012) Int J Eat Disord 45:657
37. Stunkard A, Messick S (1985) J Psychosom Res 29:71
38. Wojcicki T, White S, McAuley E (2009) J Gerontol Ser B, Psychol Sci Soc Sci 64B:33
39. Drasic L, Giabbanelli P (2015) Can J Diabetes 39(S1):S12
40. Giabbanelli PJ, Jackson PJ, Finegood DT (2014) Modelling the joint effect of social determinants and peers on obesity among canadian adults. Springer, Berlin Heidelberg, Berlin, Heidelberg, pp 145–160
41. Giabbanelli P, Crutzen R (2017) Comput Math Methods Med p 5742629
42. Hamid TK (2009) Thinking in circles about obesity, 2nd edn. Springer
43. Rahmandad H (2014) PLOS ONE 9(12):1
44. Canada S (2013) Population by broad age groups and sex, counts, including median age, 1921 to 201 for both sexes. http://www12.statcan.gc.ca/census-recensement/2011/dp-pd/hlt-fst/assa/Pages/highlight.cfm?TabID=3
45. Broemeling A, Watson D, Prebtani F (2008) Healthc Q 11(3):70
46. O'Donnell D, Deesomchok A, Lam YM, Guenette J, Amornputtisathaporn N, Forkert L, Webb K (2011) Chest 140(2):461
47. Ahern A, Aveyard P, Halford J, Mander A, Cresswell L, Cohn S, Suhrcke M, Marsh T, Thomson A, Jebb S (2014) BMC Public Health 14:620
48. Galobardes B, Shaw M, Lawlor D, Lynch J, Smith G (2006) J Epidemiol Commun Health 60:7
49. Kontinnen H, Mannisto S, Lahteenkorva S, Silventoinen K, Haukkala A (2010) Appetite 54:473
50. Geliebter A, Aversa A (2003) Eat Behav 3(4):341
51. Macht M, Simons G (2011) Emotion regulation and well-being, pp 281–295
52. Loureiro ML, Nayga RM (2006) Soc Sci Med 62:2458
53. Galuska D, Will J, Serdula M, Ford E (1999) JAMA 282(16):1576
54. Rose G, Khaw KT, Marmot M (2008) Rose's strategy of preventive medicine. Oxford University Press, New York, NY
55. Ahern A, Boyland E, Jebb S, Cohn S (2013) Ann Family Med 11(3):251
56. Bean M, Stewart K, Olbrisch M (2008) J Clin Psychol Med Settings 15(3):214
57. Forman-Hoffman V, Little A, Wahls T (2006) BMC Family Pract 7(35)
58. Fraenkel L, McGraw S (2007) J Gen Int Med 22(5):614
59. Mead N, Bower P (2000) Soc Sci Med 51(7):1087
60. Perri M, Nezu A, Viegener B (1992) Improving the long-term management of obesity: theory, research, and clinical guidelines. Wiley
61. Cooper Z, Fairburn C, Hawker D (2004) Cognitive-behavioural treatment of obesity: a clinicians guide. The Guilford Press, New York, NY
62. Giabbanelli PJ, Adams J, Pillutla VS (2016) Feasibility and framing of interventions based on public support: leveraging text analytics for policymakers. Springer International Publishing, Cham, pp 188–200

Part V
Challenges and New Frontiers

The Cornerstones of Smart Home Research for Healthcare

Kevin Bouchard, Jianguo Hao, Bruno Bouchard, Sébastien Gaboury,
Mohammed Tarik Moutacalli, Charles Gouin-Vallerand,
Hubert Kenfack Ngankam, Hélène Pigot and Sylvain Giroux

Abstract The aging of the world population has a strong impact on the world wide health care expenditure and is especially significant for countries providing free health care services to their population. One of the consequences is the increase in semi-autonomous persons requiring to be placed in specialized long term care centers. These kinds of facilities are very costly and often not appreciated by their residents. The idea of "aging in place" or living in one's home independently is a key solution to counter the impact of institutionalization. It can decrease the costs for the institutions while maximizing the quality of life of the individuals. However, these semi-autonomous persons require assistance during their daily life activities that professionals cannot hope to completely fill. Many envision the use of the smart home concept, a home equipped with distributed sensors and effectors, to add an assistance

K. Bouchard (✉) · J. Hao · B. Bouchard · S. Gaboury
LIARA Lab, Université du Québec à Chicoutimi, Chicoutimi, Canada
e-mail: Kevin.Bouchard@uqac.ca

J. Hao
e-mail: Jiango.Hao1@uqac.ca

B. Bouchard
e-mail: Bruno.Bouchard@uqac.ca

S. Gaboury
e-mail: Sebastien.Gaboury@uqac.ca

M. T. Moutacalli
Université du Québec à Rimouski, Rimouski, Canada
e-mail: mohamedtarik_moutacalli@uqar.ca

C. Gouin-Vallerand
LICEF Research Center, TÉLUQ, Montréal, Canada
e-mail: charles.gouin-vallerand@teluq.ca

H. Kenfack Ngankam · H. Pigot · S. Giroux
DOMUS Lab, Université de Sherbrooke, Sherbrooke, Canada
e-mail: Hubert.Kenfack.Ngankam@usherbrooke.ca

H. Pigot
e-mail: Helene.Pigot@usherbrooke.ca

S. Giroux
e-mail: Sylvain.Giroux@usherbrooke.ca

© Springer International Publishing AG, part of Springer Nature 2018
P. J. Giabbanelli et al. (eds.), *Advanced Data Analytics in Health*, Smart Innovation,
Systems and Technologies 93, https://doi.org/10.1007/978-3-319-77911-9_11

layer for these semi-autonomous populations. Still, despite years of research, there are several challenges to overcome in order to implement the smart home dream. This chapter positions itself as an easy to read introduction for readers unfamiliar with the challenges faced by computer science researchers regarding this difficult endeavor. It aims to walk the reader through the cornerstones of smart home research for health care.

Keywords Smart home · Aging in place · Activity recognition · Activity prediction · Context awareness · Dynamic service

1 Introduction

In western societies, the aging of the population is expected to have a major impact on the economy, society, and health care system over the next 30 years. This new reality can be considered as the most significant social transformation of the twenty-first century, with implications to many sectors, especially in the field of housing [53]. World Health Organisation (WHO) defines active aging as the process of optimizing opportunities for health, participation and security in order to enhance quality of life as people age [55]. Although aging does not necessarily imply illness or disability, the risk of both does increase. Despite these risks, elders usually prefer aging at home rather being placed in long term care facilities [35]. Therefore, the main consequence of an aging population is that affordable senior housing with supportive services remain a key component to the worlds long-term care continuum. Nevertheless, many challenges arise if one wants to provide adequate services to these semi-autonomous populations. The fundamental question is then how to provide cost-efficient adapted care services at home to a growing number of elders considering the increasing staff shortage in the field of health care [8].

Technology can certainly be part of the solution to this challenge. From that perspective, the home environment could be adapted using intelligent technologies and sensors to offset cognitive and physical deficiencies, to provide assistance and guidance to the resident, and to support the caregivers [9]. This vision of the future, which has now become a reality, originated in 1988 at the Xerox Palo Alto Research Center (PARC), resulting in the work entitled "The Computer for the 21st Century" by Mark Weiser [54]. From the early 1990s, a large community of scientists developed around this specific research niche [8], actively seeking technological solutions for these very human problems by employing such concepts as ubiquitous sensors, ambient intelligence (AMI) and assistive technologies to keep people in their homes. This concept took the form of what we now know under the name of "smart homes" [45]. A smart home is a home extended with pervasive technologies to provide relevant assistance services to its residents [18]. In our context, the aim is to increase autonomy, enhance comfort, improve sense of safety, and optimize resource management for both the elders and the caregivers [25, 40]. For instance, a smart home could support elders in their activities of daily living while informing caregivers when help is required. Thanks to a complex infrastructure of sensors and reasoning, a home becomes aware of what is going on, and if needed, it can provide near real-time advices for completing activities safely.

The goal of this chapter is to introduce the reader to the research on smart home for assistance to semi-autonomous population. On one hand, this particular context offer several opportunities, but, on the other hand, it creates challenges that must be solved in order for the technology to gain traction. While it is by nature a very multi-disciplinary field of research, this chapter contributes by reviewing the cornerstones in research on smart home for health care from a computer science point of view [5]. This chapter should not be seen as a literature review on these challenges, but as mandatory work to understand why there are still so many research teams working on these subjects despite all the progress that as been made in the recent state-of-the-art. Therefore, the remaining headwinds are described assuming the reader has a basic knowledge of each of the topics discussed in the chapter. Finally, as the reader will see in the discussion section, there are several other issues with smart homes for assistance that are beyond the scope of this chapter (e.g. the business model), but are nonetheless important.

In the next section, the reader is introduced to the foundations of smart home research and the key fundamental elements are described. Thereafter, the chapter reviews the three main challenges in developing smart homes. The first challenge is how to recognize the ongoing activities of daily living of the person. The second challenge is how to learn, predict, and adapt over time using historical data. The third is how to develop dynamic services delivery in order to adequately provide assistance when needed to the resident. Finally, the chapter concludes with a discussion on other challenges in smart homes and with some perspectives on the future directions of research.

2   Foundations of Smart Homes

Smart homes represent a promising solution to enable aging at home in our society. However, for the technology to be adopted, the services it provides must be reliable and the assistance must be relevant for the end users [41]. Thus, multiple challenges arise in the development of smart homes. They range from hardware that must be reliable (through self monitoring and *ad hoc* networking [46]) to software and AI algorithms that must infer relevant context-aware assistance opportunities. Trying to cover all of these issues would require a complete book on the subject, but, in computer science, three issues are particularly important for the technology to work. Before discussing them into details, it is important to define the concept of smart home we adopt and to go through a brief history of the work done in the last few decades.

2.1   A Pervasive Infrastructure for Ambient Intelligence

In a smart home, a pervasive infrastructure relies on sensors and actuators placed at strategic locations. Services to residents are then personalized based on their needs and requirements [23, 54]. The sensors gather low-level information on actions performed in the home: movement detectors sense human presence; contact sensors inform when doors are open or closed; pressure sensors are triggered when one lies on a bed; flow meters monitor when the toilet is flushed or when the dishwasher is started; RFID readers identify and track tagged objects [20]. Such low-level information can then be analyzed to infer the progress of high-level activities (see Sect. 3), those performed correctly, erroneous ones, and even those not performed at all. Assistance can then be provided, if necessary, helping people to complete their activities, correcting errors, preventing risks, or sending alerts to caregivers (see Sect. 5). Such assistance opportunities are highly dependent on the quality and the granularity of the information inferred from the low-level sensors [15].

In the literature, research on smart homes as well as their services and objectives take many forms. The MIT's Smart Room is considered to be the first intelligent housing laboratories to offer assistance services [39]. It was used mainly to develop a set of computer programs necessary for the recognition of facial expressions and gestures. The Adaptive House [37], from Mozer et al., is a self-programmable house that adapts to the individual's daily routine. Another similar project, the Aware Home [32], aims to produce an environment capable of understanding the parameters and the properties of the housing facility and the place where different activities of the inhabitant are carried out to better take into account the activities of everyday life in a habitat. The CASAS smart home [17] is modeled as an intelligent agent that has goals, perceives and pilots its environment. Its objective is to enable aging in place while improving the comfort of its residents and reducing the energy requirement. The LIARA [11] and DOMUS [40] smart homes were first designed to play the role of a cognitive orthotics for populations afflicted with a cognitive impairment. They both aimed at high granularity activity assistance as opposed to other projects, such as GatorTech [26], which supports residents at a high level of abstraction (by providing health related metrics or a decision support system for example).

There is no commonly accepted definition of what a smart home is in the literature, and very often, the challenges are subjectively defined by the researchers through the goal they aim to achieve with the technology. In our case, we adopt the point of view of smart homes for fine grained assistance in the daily life of the resident (e.g. helping the resident to complete a recipe or assisting with the realization of a rehabilitation program); not only as a tool to ensure security or measure the resident's health status. It is important for the reader to understand this in order to understand the challenges identified in the state-of-the-art that are described through this chapter.

3 Activity Recognition for Ambient Assistance

Recognizing human activities in smart homes plays an essential role for the purpose of assistance. With pervasive sensor networks and ambient intelligence technologies [17], sensor-based smart homes may analyze ambient changes caused by human behaviors, and provide appropriate services, supports, feedbacks, preventive warnings or interventions for their residents at the right time by means of context-aware applications [9]. An *activity recognition module* is an inference system that tries to find, among all defined activities models, the one that best explains the detected actions, which are, themselves, inferred from the set of low-level sensors (Fig. 1). Despite efforts over the past decades, activity recognition remains a challenging task for the scientific community due to the particular characteristics and the flexible designs of smart homes. Some of the most important difficulties faced by researchers are described below.

Diversified Data Types. To monitor and capture ambient conditions as comprehensively as possible, heterogeneous sensors are ubiquitously deployed in smart homes. Because of no uniform specification, captured sensor data may be discrete, continuous, nominal (categorical), binary, ordinal or numeric [10]. Thus, it is necessary to choose appropriate methods to handle these heterogeneous data.

Large-Scale Data. In smart homes built on a decentralized architecture, devices and sensors mutually communicate and exchange information all the time. Ambient changes are memorized as multi-dimensional data. The temporal and sequential data is usually noisy and numerous. On this account, an activity recognition program not only requires efficient methods to handle large-scale data, but also effective preprocessing such as feature selection to reduce dimensionality [27]. Moreover, very often the data is too big to be stored permanently and thus the algorithms may need to be able to work with incomplete history or with streams of data.

Unreliable Data Source. For many unpredictable events, captured sensor data is not always reliable. The sensors' values may be anomalous due to misreading,

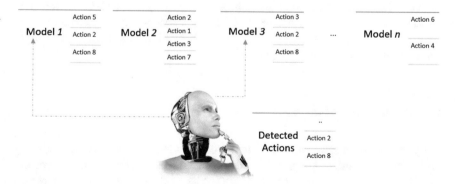

Fig. 1 Activity recognition system

insensitivity or failure of sensors themselves [46]. Moreover, the situations of signal overlapping or mutual interference could not be totally avoided. In the case of multiple residents, the values are also easy to be affected by one or more residents. Besides, even if all the information collected are reliable, there is always redundant data caused by frequent sampling and repeatedly triggering, dispensable data caused by unnecessary sensors, or reversible contextual order due to loose causal constraints between two sequential data.

Various Behavioral Patterns. Human behaviors are basically performed in sequential and complex ways. Thus, captured sensor data is usually continuous without clear boundaries. Consequently, it is difficult to segment sensor data by activities in the recognition process. Moreover, an activity could have many particular ways to be achieved. The ways here are defined as patterns (or sequences of sensor events). Based on different living habits or personal preferences, an activity could have multiple behavioral patterns describing it.

Various Granularity. The activities of daily living (ADLs) can be classified as basic or instrumental [30]. Basic activities refer to essential self-maintaining tasks like feeding, dressing, or grooming. However, these activities are usually mutually exclusive, and difficult to assist adequately due to few component actions and short execution times. In contrast, the instrumental ones involve more actions, and need more planning and interactions. Most of the state-of-the-art literature focus on recognizing the ADLs on a broad abstract level (e.g. cooking). This coarsely grained recognition does not allow for multiple assistance opportunities [15]. This granularity problem, in the authors' opinion, is the number one limitation of current activity recognition methods.

Multiple Activities. When a resident tries to perform more than one activity over a period of time, there are three alternative ways: sequential, interleaved, or concurrent modes [47]. The method of discrimination is to analyze the composition of sequences, and the contexts among sensor data. Additionally, the complexity of recognition increases when there are multiple residents in smart environments. All the residents could be performing their own activities in parallel with the three aforementioned modes, or cooperate to accomplish joint activities with other residents. Then, the captured data may belong to one or more residents, and it is hard to determine which resident triggered a sensor event. Figure 2 demonstrates few of these scenarios and their inherent complexity.

3.1 Principal Solutions

It is challenging to summarize the literature on human activity recognition, especially since the best techniques depends on several factors that cannot be readily compared (e.g. ADLs granularity, type of sensors used, online versus offline recognition, etc.). They are often separated into two families: data-driven approaches and

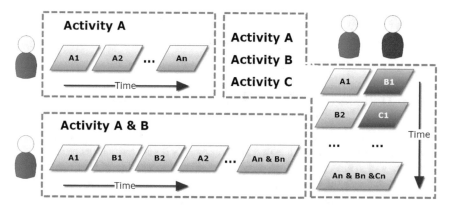

Fig. 2 Various ADLs scenarios and there timeline

knowledge driven approaches [15]. Mainstream data-driven solutions for activity recognition use both statistical and probabilistic reasoning such as hidden Markov models (HMMs), conditional random fields (CRFs), Bayesian networks, and their variations [4, 14]. These methods work fairly well in the field. However, reliable transition probabilities and emission matrices depend on a large amount of training data having stable probability distributions [10]. As a consequence, their results are sensitive to unbalanced distributions [24]. Researchers have tried in the past to deal with such imbalance, for example in [21]. Most of the other solutions are driven by prior domain knowledge, predefined rules or logic expressions [56]. Typical ones are usually to build ontological models based on knowledge representation languages such as the Web Ontology Language Description Logic (OWL-DL), or customized public ontologies [43]. Nevertheless, the definition, customization, maintenance, and extension of knowledge-driven models normally need significant artificial costs because they require human interventions from domain experts [16].

Given this weakness of knowledge-driven methods, some methods try to automatically generate the knowledge or the rules. They emphasize the analysis of occurrences and similarities about particular contexts or sensor events inside sequences. With this objective, they summarize and reuse historical data to look for regular patterns or hidden correlations in order to match new patterns with previous similar cases. The frequent pattern mining is the main solution to discover and group similar patterns [42]. Recently, several authors [24] have proposed an inference engine based on formal concept analysis that maximizes and extracts ontological correlations between patterns, and then clusters them to construct a graphical knowledge base. Sometimes, knowledge-driven methods use the data-driven ones as extensions to form a hybrid approach [6, 44].

To conclude, no method to this day exist that could completely solve the difficulties regarding activity recognition in smart homes. Knowledge driven approaches are complex to build and are time consuming. *Ad Hoc* algorithms are often working better than general algorithms, but they are not reusable. Probabilistic and statistical methods require a lot of historic data and pure machine learning methods provide a form of blackbox models difficult to exploit in assistance systems.

4 Learning and Predicting the Habits over Time

As discussed in the previous section, the activity recognition system is a core component of the artificial intelligence of a smart home for health care. It is one of the cornerstones which are necessary to provide the adequate assistance services. In order to be fully operational, however, the smart home should include other functionalities aiming to address several additional problems which go beyond the normal timeline:

- What if the observed person is performing an activity that does not exist in our activities models, or performing it in a very different way?
- What happens if the observed person is unable to start a required activity, such as taking medication?

These problems refer to a complementary task to the activity recognition which is often called the *prediction step* [34]. This part of the system is to adopt a dynamic and personalized approach for creating activities models; a task well-suited for machine learning techniques. With such a module, the system could be able to remind the assisted person to start an activity in case of forgetfulness or inability to initiate it.

4.1 Emergence of Machine Learning

The first activity recognition systems avoided the creation of activities models by assuming that they already had the complete library of activities in their knowledge bases [31]. However, creating such a large database containing all possible activities, with all different ways to perform them, is impossible to scale, slow and costly in human resources. On the other hand, machine learning algorithms are well-suited for finding frequent sequences [50]. If we consider the activities as ordered sequence of activated sensors, using a history log of activated sensors the task of creating the activities' models can be automated such as in [12, 28].

Besides the creation of activities models, machine learning techniques can also capture very useful information that can improve classical activity recognition. For example, the usual starting time or ending time of an activity could be learned. From the model on the Fig. 1, with the detected actions 2 and 8, the activity recognition system still could not choose between model 1 and 3. However, if we know that activity 1 is usually performed at 10 a.m., activity 3 at 6 p.m. and the current time is 9:55 a.m., activity 1 will be chosen because it is more likely. This is obviously a very simple example, but the idea can be used for more complex scenarios.

Average time between two adjacent sensors of an activity can also be very useful. It can help decide activating an effector, for offering assistance, when this time is exceeded without detecting the activation of the second sensor. It can also help differentiate activities. For instance, consider two sensing events produced by a smart power analyzer: ON (for boiling water), followed by OFF five minutes later. Then it can be inferred that the activity being performed is making coffee or tea. However, if the events are separated by more than ten minutes, maybe an error was made or maybe the person is doing something else. The time can also be used to check whether an action of another activity can be performed before the activation of the second sensor (cross-linked activities).

4.2 Activity Prediction

As we discussed in the previous section, the goal of a good activity recognition systems for smart home assistance is to be able to recognize the ADLs with a high granularity in order to provide useful assistance services. Therefore, ideal activity recognition systems should be able to detect actions in order to infer the activity being performed. If a prediction stage does not precede the recognition one, the system cannot assist the home occupant when no action is detected. This may happen to everyone, especially elderly people who forget to perform an important activity, or cognitively impaired patients who are even susceptible to initiation errors which prevent them from starting an activity [7].

Activity prediction stage can be designed in different manners. In [28], Allen temporal relations [3] were used to produce some rules of the kind: activity 1 precede activity 2, etc. So, when activity 1 is detected, activity 2 is predicted to be next. In contrast, in [36], starting times of each activity of each day are organized as a time series and techniques like ARIMA and VAR are used to predict activities starting times for the next day. Using time series for predicting activities starting times helps not only in assisting the smart home occupant even when no action is detected, but it also accelerates activity recognition by reducing the number of activities models that will be considered during activity recognition. Referring back to our previous example, at 9:55 a.m., model 3 will not be considered among activities models (its starting time is far different from current time), which means less comparisons and a faster activity recognition system. In order to reduce the number of considered activities models, activity prediction may also use spatial data, as in [13]. Knowing the smart home's location excludes activities that occur outside that location. For example, if the resident is in the bedroom, it can be assumed that he is not taking a shower.

When humans are observing another person performing some actions, they spontaneously use various kind of information in order to assist the person adequately (e.g., time, location, tools used). In the same way, the ambient agent must use all types of data that can be obtained for a robust and real-time assistance system in a smart home. Enriched by this information, a prediction system can further improve the ability of the assistive system to help the resident.

5 Dynamic Service Delivery for an Active Resident

Smart homes include a large range of interaction devices, from computers, televisions and smart phones to embedded display in Internet-of-Things (IoT) devices. Each of these types of devices represents an opportunity to interact with the residents, for specific tasks (e.g. a fridge) or polyvalent ones (e.g. smart phones). To assist the resident in their smart home, or across their daily living activities outside of the home, context-aware and intelligent systems are required to provide active assistive services, depending on their current whereabouts, their profile (e.g. preferences, physical or cognitive limitations), the context and the available devices. A context-aware system is a system that has the ability to capture, model and use specific information about the environment surrounding the system, such as location, time, user profile, environments topology [19].

5.1 Desirable Properties of a Service Delivery System

An intelligent service delivery system allows dynamic, fast and adapted service deployment toward the users in the environment, based on the context of the environment, and takes into account different constraints such as the users' capabilities and their preferences. We view the main goal of a service delivery system as supporting the deployment of assistive services into the smart environments for other smart systems like activity recognition or error and failure recognition systems [47]. These systems use the service delivery functionalities by sending a deployment or an activation request to the service delivery system, by supplying the information related to the assistance that needs to be deployed: Which user? Which software? What are the software needs? Is there a specific zone of the environment that is targeted by the assistance request? What is the current user activity? Is it a low priority or a high priority service delivery? and so on. To do so, directive or recommended based service delivery approaches are available, depending of several factors: context, type of services to deploy, user profiles, type of devices, etc. There are several challenges toward building a context-aware service delivery system.

Complexity of the Environment. The complexity of smart environments with their heterogeneous devices, specific configurations, and the important quantity of information to process, turn the service delivery into a serious challenge when real-time and context precision are some of the systems requirements [48]. Adaptable platforms are required to support the *ad hoc* use of devices that were not planned for at the design level [1]. Ideally, any device should be supported and their specific requirements should be downloaded dynamically in order to provide guidance to the system for adjustment. Deploying systems that provide a *plug and play* way to provide service delivery, by managing all the configurations and device heterogeneities, can help to a broader deployment and usage of the smart environment technologies.

Integration of the Service Delivery System. Another challenge is about the integration of a context-aware service delivery system into a smart home. These systems, made to be highly flexible, can be complex and difficult to adapt to specific software [38]. However, the service delivery system plays the role of a *glue* inside a smart home; it carries information between all the other systems and the end user. Since no standard exists to communicate the information between smart home systems (regarding information formatting especially), this task can be very arduous.

5.2 Current and Past Efforts for Service Delivery

Numerous efforts have been made in the development of platforms to support the delivery of assistance or services in the context of smart homes and ambient intelligence. The first works to describe the service delivery in smart environments were published around the beginning of this century, such as the Microsoft's `EasyLiving` project [49]. In this project, the researchers proposed the `EasyLiving Geometric Model` (EZLGM), a mechanism that determines which devices, in a given environment, can be used by a user during human-machine interactions and help in the selection of the right devices. The EZLGM models the relation (with measurements which describe the position and the orientation of an entity's coordinate frame) between entities, then uses geometrical transformations to determine if there is a relationship between entities.

More recently, Syed et al. [51] proposed an architecture for organizing autonomous software processes among devices of a smart space. To do this, the authors proposed the use of an intelligent system which is based on a knowledge representation of the system entities divided into four types of data: recipes, capabilities, rules, and properties. At the arrival of a service delivery in a smart space, the system compares the context of the query with the contexts of basic recipes. If the conditions in the recipe are checked and there is the presence of a device that can fulfill the requirements, a deployment policy is implemented.

In these previous systems, it is possible to impose the services to users or recommend services with different techniques. Using the context-aware models and recommendation algorithms to provide services or contents, Adomavicius et al. [2] was one of the first to propose context-aware recommender system which works on integrating contextual information in a multidimensional analysis of the users' preferences (in collaborative filtering) depending of the period of the day. Other works have been done on location-based recommender systems. For instance, Levandoski et al. [33] proposed a solution based on three types of location ratings (spatial rating for non-spatial items, non-spatial rating for spatial items, and spatial rating for spatial items). This approach is similar to the work of Adomavicius, where they used four-tuples or five-tuples to specify the ratings and used multidimensional analysis techniques to compare ratings, but with an extended definition of the context.

Finally, the `Tyche` project [22] is a distributed middleware that is made to be deployed on device nodes within smart homes and to allow the automatic deployment and management of software on environment nodes based on the device capabilities and users' profile. To automatically manage the service delivery, the middleware analyzes the contextual information of the environments, provided by the different device nodes and sensor networks, to find which devices would fit best for hosting the services. To fulfill the service delivery, Tyche's reasoning mechanism uses four main contextual elements to deploy services toward the users: the profiles of devices in the environment, the logical configuration of the environment, the user profiles, and the software profiles. Finally, all these components are present in the smart environments at different (or not) locations and are related to contextual zones. Therefore, the goal of the Tyche service delivery mechanism is to manage all this information and find the optimal organization scheme to provide the services.

6 Discussion

As we discussed in the introduction, the smart home dream is now almost three decades old. Despite this fact, most of the smart home initiatives for health care never leave the ground of the research laboratories. There are still difficult problems arising in computer science to build an artificial intelligence for assistive smart homes. Three sections were dedicated to the three most important challenges in this chapter (Sects. 3–5). However, we selected other issues that are linked to the core problems of smart home research, and summarized them below. The authors hope to provide the readers with opportunities to further explore the topic of smart homes for aging in place with these selected issues.

6.1 Heterogeneous Hardware

A wide spectrum of equipment types and manufacturers are available, leading to much heterogeneity between hardware, networks, and applications [29]. Since a single manufacturer cannot typically address all needs and contexts, many technologies have to coexist and must cooperate. The software architecture must then allow to integrate such an eclectic variety of equipments, protocols, and services to ensure transparency with respect to information exchange, applications and services. This situation is also known as the *vertical handover* [57].

6.2 Ethics

Social and ethical concerns result from ubiquitous technology within smart homes [52]. First, technological dependencies may impede individuals instead of fostering autonomy. Relying too much on assistance may lead to withdraw oneself from completing activities on their own, expecting the smart home to compensate their deficits. Smart home assistance could also undermine an elder's freedom by offering and even choosing only specific solutions. Finally, surveillance can put privacy at risk. Seamless integration and ubiquity of sensors can affect one's ability to detect their presence and knowing exactly what is monitored or not. Moreover huge memory capacity of computers could allow to set up surveillance that could persist across time and space, more than necessary.

6.3 The Stakeholders' Dilemma

Finally, one very difficult issue regarding smart home for health care is very rarely discussed. The stakeholders' dilemma refer to the disruptive nature of these new technologies. There are currently no business models for the smart home and it is far from clear who is going to pay to implement the smart homes to assist the elders. Will it be the government through public health spending? Insurances? Or should it be left to private corporation? An open-mind must be kept regarding the business model.

7 Conclusion

This chapter presented the cornerstones of smart home research for health care with a specific emphasis on computer science difficulties regarding the construction of an artificial intelligence in smart homes. Smart homes are a challenging endeavor, and while the literature has progressed a lot on all of the topics presented, there are still several issues to overcome in order to implement the smart home dream. In particular, the cornerstones of smart home research for healthcare are the activity recognition, the learning and the prediction of the behaviors over time, and the context aware service delivery. The AI discussed in this paper was, however, the ideal one. The lack of ideal solutions does not mean that smart homes could not prove useful in the present. Smaller, simpler smart homes can be implemented to provide services to semi-autonomous residents, provided an adequate business model is found. Future work should address this important question.

References

1. Abowd G, Dey A, Brown P, Davies N, Smith M, Steggles P (1999) Towards a better understanding of context and context-awareness. In: Handheld and ubiquitous computing. Springer, pp 304–307

2. Adomavicius G, Tuzhilin A (2015) Context-aware recommender systems. In: Recommender systems handbook. Springer, pp 191–226
3. Allen JF, Ferguson G (1994) Actions and events in interval temporal logic. J Logic Comput 4(5):531–579
4. Amiribesheli M, Benmansour A, Bouchachia A (2015) A review of smart homes in healthcare. J Ambient Intell Humaniz Comput 6(4):495–517
5. Augusto JC, Nugent CD (2006) Smart homes can be smarter. In: Designing smart homes. Springer, pp 1–15
6. Azkune G, Almeida A, López-de Ipiña D, Chen L (2015) Extending knowledge-driven activity models through data-driven learning techniques. Expert Syst Appl 42(6):3115–3128
7. Baum C, Edwards DF (1993) Cognitive performance in senile dementia of the alzheimers type: the kitchen task assessment. Am J Occup Therapy 47(5):431–436
8. Blackman S, Matlo C, Bobrovitskiy C, Waldoch A, Fang ML, Jackson P, Mihailidis A, Nygård L, Astell A, Sixsmith A (2016) Ambient assisted living technologies for aging well: a scoping review. J Intell Systs 25(1):55–69
9. Bouchard B (2017) Smart technologies in healthcare. CRC press, Taylor & Francis
10. Bouchard K, Bergeron F, Giroux S (2017) Applying data mining in smart home. In: Smart technologies in healthcare, p 146
11. Bouchard K, Bouchard B, Bouzouane A (2012) Guidelines to efficient smart home design for rapid AI prototyping: a case study. In: Proceedings of the 5th international conference on pervasive technologies related to assistive environments. ACM, p 29
12. Bouchard K, Bouzouane A, Bouchard B (2013) Discovery of topological relations for spatial activity recognition. In: 2013 IEEE symposium on computational intelligence and data mining (CIDM). IEEE, pp 73–80
13. Bouchard K, Fortin-Simard D, Lapalu J, Gaboury S, Bouzouane A, Bouchard B (2015) Unsupervised spatial data mining for smart homes. In: 2015 IEEE international conference on data mining workshop (ICDMW). IEEE, pp 1433–1440
14. Chen L, Hoey J, Nugent CD, Cook DJ, Yu Z (2012) Sensor-based activity recognition. IEEE Trans Syst Man, Cybern Part C (Applications and Reviews) 42(6):790–808
15. Chen L, Khalil I (2011) Activity recognition: approaches, practices and trends. In: Activity recognition in pervasive intelligent, environments, pp 1–31
16. Chen L, Nugent CD, Wang H (2012) A knowledge-driven approach to activity recognition in smart homes. IEEE Trans Knowl Data Eng 24(6):961–974
17. Cook DJ, Augusto JC, Jakkula VR (2009) Ambient intelligence: technologies, applications, and opportunities. Pervasive Mobile Comput 5(4):277–298
18. Demiris G, Rantz MJ, Aud MA, Marek KD, Tyrer HW, Skubic M, Hussam AA (2004) Older adults' attitudes towards and perceptions of smart home technologies: a pilot study. Med Inform Internet Med 29(2):87–94
19. Dey AK, Abowd GD, Salber D (2001) A conceptual framework and a toolkit for supporting the rapid prototyping of context-aware applications. Human Comput Interact 16(2):97–166
20. Fortin-Simard D, Bilodeau J-S, Bouchard K, Gaboury S, Bouchard B, Bouzouane A (2015) Exploiting passive RFID technology for activity recognition in smart homes. IEEE Intell Syst 30(4):7–15
21. Giabbanelli PJ, Peters JG (2015) An algebraic approach to combining classifiers. Procedia Comput Sci 51:1545–1554
22. Gouin-Vallerand C, Abdulrazak B, Giroux S, Dey AK (2013) A context-aware service provision system for smart environments based on the user interaction modalities. J Ambient Intell Smart Environ 5(1):47–64
23. Hansmann U, Merk L, Nicklous MS, Stober T (2003) Pervasive computing: the mobile world. Springer Science & Business Media
24. Hao J, Bouzouane A, Gaboury S (2017) Complex behavioral pattern mining in non-intrusive sensor-based smart homes using an intelligent activity inference engine. J Reliab Intell Environ. pp 1–18
25. Harper R (2006) Inside the smart home. Springer Science & Business Media

26. Helal S, Mann W, El-Zabadani H, King J, Kaddoura Y, Jansen E (2005) The GatorTech smart house: a programmable pervasive space. Computer 38(3):50–60
27. Hinton GE, Salakhutdinov RR (2006) Reducing the dimensionality of data with neural networks. Science 313(5786):504–507
28. Jakkula V, Cook DJ (2007) Mining sensor data in smart environment for temporal activity prediction. In: Poster session at the ACM SIGKDD, San Jose, CA
29. Kamilaris A, Pitsillides A, Trifa V (2011) The smart home meets the web of things. Int J Ad Hoc Ubiquitous Comput 7(3):145–154
30. Katz S (1983) Assessing self-maintenance: activities of daily living, mobility, and instrumental activities of daily living. J Am Geriatr Soc 31(12):721–727
31. Kautz HA, Allen JF (1986) Generalized plan recognition. In: AAAI, vol 86, p 5
32. Kientz JA, Patel SN, Jones B, Price E, Mynatt ED, Abowd GD (2008) The Georgia tech aware home. In: CHI'08 Extended abstracts on human factors in computing systems. ACM, pp 3675–3680
33. Levandoski JJ, Sarwat M, Eldawy A, Mokbel MF (2012) LARS: a location-aware recommender system. In: 2012 IEEE 28th international conference on data engineering (ICDE). IEEE, pp 450–461
34. Li K, Fu Y (2014) Prediction of human activity by discovering temporal sequence patterns. IEEE Trans Pattern Anal Mach Intell 36(8):1644–1657
35. Marek KD, Rantz MJ (2000) Aging in place: a new model for long-term care. Nurs Adm Q 24(3):1–11
36. Moutacalli MT, Bouchard K, Bouzouane A, Bouchard B (2014) Activity prediction based on time series forcasting. In: AAAI workshop on artificial intelligence applied to assistive technologies and smart environments (ATSE 14)
37. Mozer M (2004) Lessons from an adaptive house. In: Smart environments: technologies, protocols, and applications. Wiley
38. Parra J, Hossain MA, Uribarren A, Jacob E, El Saddik A (2009) Flexible smart home architecture using device profile for web services: a peer-to-peer approach. Int J Smart Home 3(2):39–56
39. Pentland AP (1996) Smart rooms. Sci Am 274(4):68–76
40. Pigot H, Lussier-Desrochers D, Bauchet J, Giroux S, Lachapelle Y (2008) A smart home to assist in recipe completion. Technol Aging, Assist Technol Res Ser 21:35–42
41. Rashidi P, Cook DJ (2009) Keeping the resident in the loop: adapting the smart home to the user. IEEE Trans Syst Man Cybern Part A: Syst Humans 39(5):949–959
42. Rashidi P, Cook DJ, Holder LB, Schmitter-Edgecombe M (2011) Discovering activities to recognize and track in a smart environment. IEEE Trans Knowl Data Eng 23(4):527–539
43. Riboni D, Bettini C (2011) OWL 2 modeling and reasoning with complex human activities. Pervasive Mobile Comput 7(3):379–395
44. Riboni D, Sztyler T, Civitarese G, Stuckenschmidt H (2016) Unsupervised recognition of interleaved activities of daily living through ontological and probabilistic reasoning. In: Proceedings of the 2016 ACM international joint conference on pervasive and ubiquitous computing. ACM, pp 1–12
45. Ricquebourg V, Menga D, Durand D, Marhic B, Delahoche L, Loge C (2006) The smart home concept: our immediate future. In: 2006 1st IEEE international conference on e-learning in industrial electronics. IEEE, pp 23–28
46. Robles RJ, Kim TH (2010) Applications, systems and methods in smart home technology: A. Int J Adv Sci Technol 15
47. Roy P, Bouchard B, Bouzouane A, Giroux S (2009) A hybrid plan recognition model for Alzheimer's patients: interleaved-erroneous dilemma. Web Intell Agent Syst Int J 7(4):375–397
48. Satyanarayanan M (2001) Pervasive computing: vision and challenges. IEEE Pers Commun 8(4):10–17
49. Shafer S, Krumm J, Brumitt B, Meyers B, Czerwinski M, Robbins D (1998) The new EasyLiving project at Microsoft research. In: Proceedings of the 1998 DARPA/NIST smart spaces workshop. pp 127–130

50. Srikant R, Vu Q, Agrawal R (1997) Mining association rules with item constraints. KDD 97:67–73
51. Syed AA, Lukkien J, Frunza R (2010). An architecture for self-organization in pervasive systems. In: Proceedings of the conference on design, automation and test in Europe. European Design and Automation Association, pp 1548–1553
52. Tavani HT (2011) Ethics and technology: controversies, questions, and strategies for ethical computing. Wiley
53. United Nations (2015) World population ageing; 2015
54. Weiser M (1995) The computer for the 21st century. Sci Am 272(3):78–89
55. World Health Organization et al (2016) Active ageing: a policy framework; 2009
56. Ye J, Stevenson G, Dobson S (2015) KCAR: a knowledge-driven approach for concurrent activity recognition. Pervasive Mobile Comput 19:47–70
57. Zekri M, Jouaber B, Zeghlache D (2012) A review on mobility management and vertical handover solutions over heterogeneous wireless networks. Comput Commun 35(17):2055–2068

Challenges and Cases of Genomic Data Integration Across Technologies and Biological Scales

Shamith A. Samarajiwa, Ioana Olan and Dóra Bihary

Abstract Current technological advancements have facilitated novel experimental methods that measure a diverse assortment of biological processes, creating a data deluge in biology and medicine. This proliferation of data sources, from large repositories and data warehouses to specialist databases that store a variety of different data types, contributing to a multitude of different file formats, have necessitated minimal data standards that describe both data and annotation. In addition to integrating at the data resource level, development of integrative computational or statistical methods that explore two or more data types or biological layers to understand their joint influence can lead to a better understanding of both normal and pathological processes. Combination of these different data-layers, in turn enables us to glean a more integrative understanding of complex biological systems. Development of integrative methods that bridge both biology and technology can provide insight into different scales of gene and genome regulation. Some of these integrative approaches and their application are explored in this chapter in the context of modern genomics.

1 Introduction

In the last couple of decades, the biomedical sciences transitioned from being small scale data producers utilising mainly reductionist approaches to becoming producers of diverse and complex "big data", enabling the exploration of a more quantitative "systems" view of life. A defining event was the development of microarray technology in the late 1980s, enabling the activity of tens of thousands of genes to be simultaneously measured [8]. This heralded the beginning of a

S. A. Samarajiwa (✉) · D. Bihary
MRC Cancer Unit, University of Cambridge, Cambridge CB2 0XZ, UK
e-mail: ss861@mrc-cu.cam.ac.uk

I. Olan
Cancer Research UK Cambridge Institute, University of Cambridge,
Cambridge CB2 0RE, UK

© Springer International Publishing AG, part of Springer Nature 2018
P. J. Giabbanelli et al. (eds.), *Advanced Data Analytics in Health*, Smart Innovation,
Systems and Technologies 93, https://doi.org/10.1007/978-3-319-77911-9_12

pivotal period in biomedicine. Consequently, this availability of high-dimensional datasets fueled the rapid development of computational algorithms and statistical data analysis methods.

The genetic material within a cell (chromosomal and mitochondrial DNA) is known as the "genome" and "genomics" is the study of genome structure and function. The Human Genome Project [28] was the international, collaborative research program that mapped the sequence of the 3.4 billion bases that constitutes human DNA. The initial human reference genome cost 2.7 billion USD, an undertaking that took more than 13 years. Sanger sequencing played a prominent role in this emergent genomics revolution and was subsequently replaced by cheaper and faster massively parallel DNA sequencing technologies. Human genomes produced by the early Illumina sequencing machines cost $300,000 USD per genome in 2006. These can now be sequenced in less than a day and cost less than $1000 USD in 2017. Due to technological advancements, next generation sequencing capacity doubles every seven months growing at a rate faster than Moore's law. Consequently, the cost of these technologies has exponentially decreased over time. Sequencing a genome for $100 USD within a few hours is a possibility in the near future [31].

The explosion of biomedical data is sustained by a mixture of next generation sequencing technologies, advances in mass spectroscopy and various high throughput cell-imaging technologies [24]. This 'omics' revolution has enabled the direct measurement of genomic, transcriptomic, translatomic, proteomic, epigenomic and metabolomic cellular information layers at both the population and single cell level. Each data type provides a distinct, partially independent and complementary view of the cellular information flow. The deluge of data being produced in biology is exemplified by the current global genomic sequencing data production, estimated at 35 petabytes per year [59]. The advent of sensor based medical devices and emergent personalised medicine technologies will also contribute to this data deluge, with zettabyte (10^9 Tb) scale data production expected by 2025. The burden of storage, management and analysis of these vastly increasing datasets is a growing obstacle to biomedical knowledge generation, requiring data science expertise with more rigorous experimental design, data-compression and storage solutions together with high performance computing and integrative analysis solutions.

Now more than ever, the application of data science methodologies to these large biological datasets to assist in the extraction, cleansing, integration, visualization, modelling and data-mining, leading to new breakthroughs in biomedicine is essential. Whilst each of these steps in the data science life cycle are important for turning data into knowledge, in this chapter we will focus on how integration of heterogeneous and complementary biomedical datasets are providing new insights into fundamental biological processes.

2 Computational Aspects

2.1 Data Repositories in Biology

Efficient integration of similar data types generated by different laboratories in different locations to optimize resource usage has been a long-standing goal in bioinformatics. With this aim, the National Centre for Biotechnology Information, an initiative of the US National Library of Medicine was founded [45] as a centralised provider of sequence data (GenBank), sequence analysis software (BLAST) and biomedical literature (PubMed). Since then, tens of thousands of specialised databases, software tools, data analysis resources (Ensembl, UCSC genome browser) and specialised sequence databases such as the Gene Expression Omnibus (GEO), ArrayExpress, Short Read Archive (SRA), European Nucleotide Archive (ENA) have emerged. Omictools, a web catalogue (https://omictools.com/) of such resources, lists over 19,300 databases and software tools [26]. Specialist biomedical publications routinely catalogue web-servers and databases (http://www. oxfordjournals.org/nar/database/c/) for biological data analysis [21]. These repositories and resources are a rich source of data for integrative endeavours.

In a seminal paper, Lincoln Stein advocated a "bioinformatics nation" built on web service technologies to integrate these data silos [58]. While RESTful web service, enabling programmatic access to data resources is becoming more prevalent, not all resource providers have adapted such technologies. BioMart (http://www.biomart.org/), which is a freely available, open source collection of federated databases, that provide uniform access to a diverse set of geographically distributed data sources is an example of a successful biomedical data integration system [57]. It provides RESTful API's for programmatic access and graphical user interfaces for web access, as well as the R/Bioconductor biomaRt package [16]. Intermine is another such system that utilizes data warehouse technologies for integration and has been adopted by the modEncode consortium [33]. Other early attempts, such as the Distributed Annotation System (DAS) [32] which allowed genomic annotations to be decentralized between third party annotators and integrated as needed by client side software has been replaced by newer technologies such as Track Hubs and Assembly Hubs. These provide access to organised genomic data and annotation on a web server that can then be integrated and explored using genome browser software. Annotation-Hubs are the R/Bioconductor (https://www.bioconductor.org/) approach, enabling collections of public and private data to be accessed for easy integration with other datasets via an uniform programmatic R interface [44].

2.2 Biomedical Data Formats and File Types

Data integration facilitates querying and computation across different data sources and data types. The two most widely used approaches for data integration include statistical integration approaches and the use of storage and retrieval technologies to logically integrate heterogeneous information. In this latter approach, data sources are stored as flat files, relational, object oriented, graph and other NoSQL databases, or in specialised data warehouses. Some of the early biological databases such as GenBank consisted of indexed flat files and semi-structured XML [4]. The use of the relational model and relational database management systems (RDBMS) such as MySQL, MariaDB or PostgreSQL enabled data to be represented in terms of tuples and grouped into relations. NoSQL database technologies such as MongoDb or CouchDb enabled indexing and fast searching of document stores. Resource description framework (RDF) formats together with the SPARQL query language can also represent linked data as triple stores, which utilize a set of three entities that encode statements about semantic relationships in the form of subject-predicate-object [11, 47]. Graph databases such as Neo4j and GraphDB excel at implementing these linked data principles first proposed by the web pioneer, Tim Berners-Lee [3].

Biomedical datasets can vary in size from a few megabytes (Mb) to many hundreds of terabytes (Tb) and exist in a variety of different formats such as text files, XML, images, binary formats, graph representations etc. Data collection and the painful process of cleansing, parsing and proofing, better known as data "munging" or "wrangling", form a time consuming part of most data science projects. According to a data science survey commissioned by a data-mining company [14], data munging accounts for 60–80% of project time. The diversity of biological open data specifications and file formats (Fasta, Fastq, Bam, Sam, Cram, bed, wiggle, GFF, GTF, vcf etc.) also creates challenges in extracting relevant information (https://genome.ucsc.edu/FAQ/FAQformat.html) needed for data integration endeavours [10]. In addition, fields such as proteomics and metabolomics have vendor specific 'black box' file formats further complicating data integration across data types. Even with increasing internet bandwidth, the extremely large file sizes or datasets with hundreds of samples (such as those from whole genome sequencing (WGS) or imaging experiments) make it difficult to move these files via the internet. Sadly, it has become common practice to ship or post hard drives containing WGS data to the relevant destination, rather than attempting to transfer these electronically [56].

2.3 Data Quality and Standards

Integrating your own datasets with relevant publicly available datasets provides opportunities for increasing the sample size and scope of analysis. Sharing datasets by submitting them to a public repository is essential in biology, and is required by most journals prior to publication. This encourages reproducible research and ensures reuse of datasets to solve new biomedical problems. However just submitting datasets to repositories does not enable efficient future usage. Detailed annotation describing experiments, samples and datasets is essential. Often issues such as bad experimental design, data quality issues, incomplete datasets and annotation are uncovered when attempting to integrate data downloaded from repositories.

Minimal reporting standards are needed, that specify what information about an experiment is captured, together with controlled vocabularies that define the terminology and provide definitions or identification of entities specified by each data type [60]. There are over 600 such content standards and web resources such as Biosharing (https://biosharing.org) that enable the discovery of these standards and the databases that implement them [42]. These standards are expected to be utilized when submitting datasets to repositories. Minimal information standards for microarrays (MIAME) [7], sequencing (MINSEQE), and proteomics (MIAPE) [41] (http://fged.org/projects/) facilitate the interpretation of experimental results unambiguously, enabling reproducibility, reuse and integration of data.

There are a number of experimental design and statistical considerations that must be taken into account when processing biological data for integration. Determining the appropriate number of technical or biological replicates required, by applying power analysis to estimate sample size for a given effect size before data generation is a necessity that is often ignored [12, 63]. Many statistical data integration methods are dependent on availability of multiple biological replicates and attempting to increase sample size post hoc will lead to biases such as batch effects.[1] Artefacts can also be introduced due to technical and experimental biases during data production and collection and must be removed before analysis. Tracking data provenance during the data processing workflow is also critical for reproducibility of integrated data. Workflow management systems such as Taverna [30], Galaxy [22] and Knime [18] are some of the tools that provide a data provenance solution. Other issues in data quality that also increase irreproducibility, include cell line misidentification [29] which lead to more than 32,000 articles reporting on wrong cells-lines, mis-genotyping and sample mix ups.

Small sample sizes, and large number of features per sample, are a common characteristic of datasets that measure properties of genes or proteins genome wide. The 'curse of dimensionality' introduced by high dimensional data, require dimensionality reduction algorithms such as principal component analysis (PCA), multidimensional scaling (MDS) and tSNE clustering. Multiple sampling of features necessitates false discovery rate correction methods. When multiple datasets are compared, as often occurs during data integration, appropriate normalization

---

[1]Batch effects are sources of technical variation that have been added to samples during handling and processing, such as when samples belonging to the same experiment are processed at different times, produced with different reagent batches, on different machines or by different people.

methods must be used [35]. Data type specific statistical methods have been developed for both batch effect removal [36] and normalization of transcriptomic data [38, 52].

3   Challenges in Biomedical Data Integration

Biomedical data is context dependent, requires detailed metadata and annotation, displays enormous complexity and heterogeneity, and can be extremely noisy due to the nature of technologies involved. They either lack data standards or have a plethora of competing standards, all of which contribute to integration problems. One of the key issues in biology that directly impacts integration is the lack of globally unique identifiers. Entities such as genes and proteins may be referred to by hundreds of synonyms making mapping and integration problematic. Genes discovered in model organism species such as fruit fly and zebrafish often have creative names ('Grim' and 'Reaper'—involved in cell death, 'Tinman'—mutants develop without a heart, 'Casanova'—mutants with two hearts, 'Spock'—mutants have pointy ears and 'Sonic hedgehog'—spiky coat etc.). When homologues of these were identified in humans and mice they were often given different names. This problem is succinctly described by the prominent biologist Michael Ashburner's quote that "a biologist would rather share their toothbrush than their gene name" [48]. The Human Gene Name Nomenclature committee (HGNC) database (https://www.genenames.org) is an attempt at assisting the use of unique gene names [62]. Genes having multiple synonyms (one fruit fly gene has over a 400) and multiple genes referred to by the same synonym often adds confusion to data integration efforts. While there have been attempts at creating synonym dictionaries, there is no comprehensive and reliable synonym mapping resource, and the proliferation of database specific gene identifiers have also exacerbated this problem.

The diversity of biomedicine has encouraged the production of a "long tail" of specialist bioinformatics resources that are not centralised, making data integration a formidable challenge. Consequently, each data type and specialist field generates a multiplicity of resources, many replicating each other, partially overlapping or presenting different viewpoints on similar data types. There are many consequences of this unregulated proliferation of biomedical resources and software applications. Some of these resources are built by those with little skill in data modeling, or user interface design [25]. Many such resources become obsolete within a short time and most often disappear altogether when their developers move on to different institutions, as often happens in academia. One study estimated that only 18% of such resources survive the test of time [43]. Availability of funding to generate such resource but not for their maintenance has also contributed to their short-lived nature. Building automated ways of keeping these resources up to date and giving ownership to users that will benefit the most by the specialist resource, often increase their longevity. Interferome, a specialist immunology related integrative data-resource initially released in 2009 is an example of this strategy [54]. It is regularly updated and maintained by an immunology research group, removing the burden of resource maintenance from the original developers.

An intentional or otherwise lack of understanding of the user requirements often leads to a plethora of data formats, schemas, APIs, and database technologies that are most often unsuited for task at hand. The emergence of similar resources with large overlap in data or functionality is also frequently observed. An example of this is the proliferation of pathway databases. Cellular information flow can be represented by biochemical pathways or networks that map protein interactions, signaling events, metabolic and regulatory interactions into graph representations. Pathguide, a resource of pathway databases (http://pathguide.org/) lists 646 such resources [1]. A search of multiple human pathway databases (such as Reactome, KEGG, Wikipathways, Pathway Commons, Ingenuity Pathway Analysis, Meta-Core^{TM} etc.) for any well-studied pathway will produce a set of results that are in disagreement with each other. This could range from slight inconsistencies to significant differences in entities and their functional connectivity. Biological pathways are fragments of cellular networks and their representation reflects knowledge biases of the groups and individuals that model them.

4 Insights into Genomic Regulation Using Integrative Approaches

4.1 Cellular Information Flow

One of the greatest challenges in biology is understanding the molecular basis of phenotypes. Perturbations in the external environment or the intracellular space can activate signal transduction events that in turn trigger transcription factor (TF) proteins. These TFs can either repress or induce the transcription of many other genes. Similarly, modifications of the epigenome[2] or changes in the chromatin[3] three-dimensional structure can affect regulatory activity of genes. The resultant flow of information and changes in components and interactions can be measured by modern 'omic' technologies. Data integration enables the joint influence of these different cellular processes to be assessed. An example workflow describing potential steps involving genomic data processing and data integration is

---

[2]The epigenome consists of a collection of chemical compounds that tell the DNA what to do. These can attach to DNA or proteins associated with DNA and regulate gene activity without changing the DNA sequence.

[3]Chromatin consists of DNA, the disk like nucleosomes that DNA spools around for efficient packaging, non-coding RNA and other DNA associated accessory proteins. When epigenomic compounds attach to chromatin, they are said to have "marked" the genome. These modifications do not change the sequence of the DNA, they change how cells use the information encoded by DNA.

shown in Fig. 1. Integrating TF binding with gene expression can identify TF direct targets. Integrating specific types of histone modifications assists in detecting different types of regulatory regions.

Similarly, integrating chromatin modifications and gene expression with chromatin interactions enable identifying chromosomal structural features such as topologically associating domains (TADs), chromatin hubs and enhancer-promoter loops that regulate gene expression (Fig. 1).

4.2 Modeling Cellular Regulomes

Data from molecular experiments enable modelling of cellular information flow into pathways. These methods usually capture a linear cascade of reactions or interactions between molecules, focusing on a specific phenotypic activity or molecular process. Even though this is a useful representation in understanding the connectivity of components, biological processes are usually not linear, and their connectivity can be more correctly represented as complex dynamic networks, with feedback or feed forward loops and crosstalk. As mentioned previously, there are many resources online to study cellular pathways, but our understanding of cellular networks is still in its infancy.

TFs bind to DNA regulatory elements and induce or repress the transcription of their target genes. These regulatory regions can be proximal to a gene (promoters), or more distal to their target genes (enhancers), and mapping these regulatory regions and TF binding events to target genes is challenging. Therefore, next generation sequencing (NGS) methods providing genome wide overviews have been developed to measure different aspects of cellular regulatory activities. One such technique, ChIP-seq (Chromatin Immunoprecipitation followed by massively parallel sequencing) enables detection of TF binding genomic regions [51]. Conversely, RNA-seq enables the measurement of gene expression by detecting RNA transcripts counts [49]. Importantly, a single regulatory region may regulate more than a single gene, and conversely a combination of different TFs may be required for the activation or repression of any single gene. Integrating TF binding to DNA with the transcription of the associated genes enables identification of TF direct target genes.

There are several integrative statistical methods available for this task, such as Rcade: R-based analysis of ChIP-seq And Differential Expression [9] and BETA: Binding and expression target analysis [61]. Rcade is implemented as an R/Bioconductor package that employs a Bayesian modelling approach. It computes the posterior probabilities of TF binding from ChIP-seq data, and the posterior probabilities of differential gene expression from transcriptomic data. After combining these, and ranking them by their log-odds scores and false discovery rate, the resultant genes can be used to identify TF direct targets. BETA on the other hand, depends on peak calling to detect TF binding sites and calculates a p-value based on

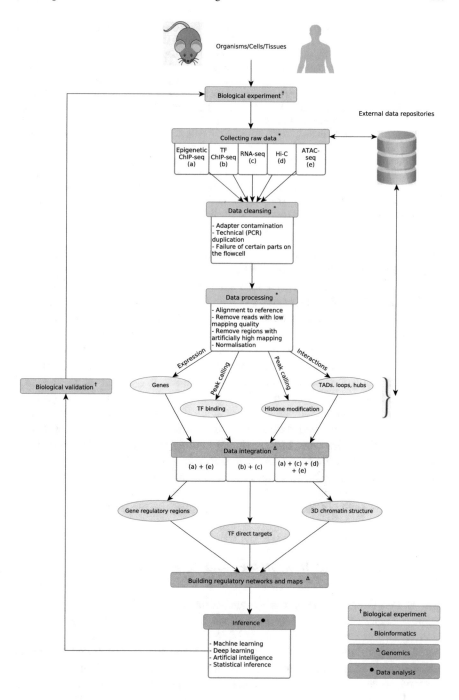

◀**Fig. 1 Data workflow for regulatory genomics**: The flow diagram explores the data processing and integration workflow for five main data types used in regulatory genomics. These data types can be either experimentally derived or downloaded from data repositories. * Data Cleansing: These sequencing datasets undergo a cleansing step, which removes noise and artefacts such as sequencing adaptors or primers, PCR duplicates and low quality reads. * Data processing: steps such as the alignment to a reference genome, removal of reads with low mapping quality, or regions with artificially high mapping is then carried out. Sample normalisation, which enables sample comparison, is performed. Finally methods for detecting biological signal (gene expression analysis, ChIP-seq peak calling, chromatin interaction detection) and integration of these biological layers to give different insights into gene and genome regulation are carried out. These include identifying TF direct targets, gene regulatory regions and resolving 3D chromatin structure. △ All of which can be used to build regulatory maps and network models. ● Application of machine learning and other statistical inference methods on these integrated datasets together with network analysis to make predictions or hypothesis generation. † Experimentally validate these hypotheses or predictions

a Kolmogorov-Smirnov test using the ranked binding and expression information to determine the most likely direct targets.

A single TF is evolutionarily constrained to regulate a finite number of target genes. This 'universe' of target genes of a particular TF is known as its 'regulome'. Once these TF direct targets have been identified, they can be utilised to build useful maps of phenotype specific gene regulation by integrating with prior biological knowledge. This could be information on subcellular localization of proteins, signaling pathways mined from various databases and protein-protein interactions integrated with regulatory interactions text-mined from the vast biomedical literature. TP53 is one of the most important tumour suppressor proteins in the cell and the TP53 gene deletion or mutation can lead to tumour formation. It is also one of the most well studied proteins with over 91,000 publications. Using the integrative process described above, TF binding and Gene expression datasets were integrated with the Bayesian method Rcade enabling the discovery of TP53 targets. Subsequently gene regulatory network maps of the TP53 Regulome (http://www.australian-systemsbiology.org/tp53/) were reverse engineered for TP53 modulated processes such as apoptosis and cellular senescence [34].

4.3   Integrating Transcriptomes and Epigenomes

The haploid (single copy) human genome contains approximately 3.4 billion base pairs packaged into 23 chromosomes. Each base pair is 0.34 nm long; therefore each diploid cell will contain 2 m of DNA [2]. Unlike bacterial DNA, which is naked, DNA of higher organisms is spooled around protein complexes known as nucleosomes. These nucleosomes are composed of pairs of 4 different types of histone proteins. Since DNA is negatively charged, it binds to the positively charged histones very tightly. This spooling around nucleosomes and the associated supercoiling processes enables the compression of the 2 m long DNA filaments into a compact 30 nm fibre. These DNA-protein filament structures are known as chromatin [39]. Electron micrographs showing spaghetti like arrangement of chromatin fibres within a nucleus mislead researchers for many years into thinking that nuclear chromatin was in a random disordered state. More recently, it's been discovered that chromosomes occupy distinct territories within the nucleus [13], and this organization promotes chromatin looping interactions that influences gene regulation [55]. The use of chromosomal conformation capture sequencing methods demonstrated that chromatin has a distinct three dimensional (3D) structure. Constrained by this 3D structure, both short and long distance chromatin interactions and local domain organization contribute to gene regulation [15].

The epigenome also has an important role in gene regulation. Chromatin can be chemically modified (methylated, phosphorylated, acetylated etc.) in at least 80 different ways; the combinatorial effect of all these modifications leads to different 'states' of the chromatin, such as active and inactive regions. ChIP-seq technology can be used to detect these chemical modifications, enabling identification of functional chromatin regions. Computational integration of regions with different modifications enable the prediction of underlying chromatin states. EpiCSeg, ChromHMM and Segway are some of the methods developed for integrative chromatin marks [17, 27, 40]. These resultant segmented regions identified by integration of different chromatin modifications can be used to define genomic regulatory regions.

4.4   Genome Architecture and Topology

We are able to characterise the dynamics of cell type specific chromatin structure in different conditions using Hi-C [37], a sequencing technology that detects interactions between different regions of the genome. A Hi-C interaction frequency matrix visualized as a heatmap is shown in Fig. 2a. Moreover, the formation of rosette like structures due to highly interacting proximal regions known as topologically associated domains (TADs) can be detected by Hi-C (Fig. 2b).

TADs demonstrate that most chromatin interactions are grouped into sets of consecutive regions on the genome with clearly delimited boundaries. Chromatin structure is affected by histone modifications (Fig. 2c), which modulates gene expression by influencing both accessibility of TFs to DNA (strong ATAC-seq signal and RNA-seq signal over the SERPINB2 gene in Fig. 2c) and by enabling chromatin interactions that enable enhancer promoter contacts (disrupted vs. single TAD in red box between condition 1 and 2 in Fig. 2b). Regulatory potential of interactions thus provide a clear approach for combining Hi-C, epigenomic and TF driven gene expression (e.g. RNA-seq) data to understand gene regulation. A few more examples of data integration in regulatory genomics are discussed below.

Isocitrate dehydrogenase (IDH) mutations with gain of function properties are a defining event in brain tumours known as gliomas. These mutant enzymes produce a metabolite that interferes with other enzyme activities and affects the epigenetic

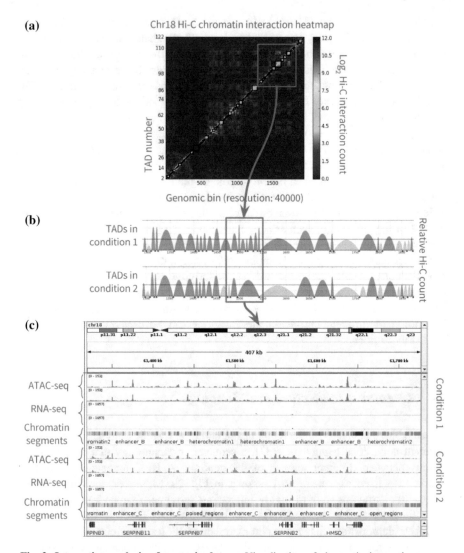

Fig. 2 Integrative analysis of genomic data: **a** Visualization of chromatin interactions as an interaction heatmap where the interaction frequencies between different regions in human chromosome 18 were determined by a Hi-C experiment. X and Y-axes show correlation of $\log_2$ interaction counts across a single chromosome in genomic bins of 40 kb resolution. **b** A region of the heatmap is expanded to visualize topologically associated domains from the same region plotted for two conditions. **c** A ~400 kb region of chromosome 18 is shown. Two replicate tracks of open chromatin regions (ATAC-seq), and gene expression (RNA-seq) in the expanded TAD region in two condition together with chromatin colour tracks are shown. These three data views show aspects of chromatin interactions that contribute to gene transcription

state of the cell. One of the effects of IDH mutations is hyper-methylation at CTCF binding sites, preventing CTCF binding at those locations. CTCF is a boundary element (insulator) of genomic regions (including TADs) and is also involved in chromatin loop formation. Using an integrative chromatin analysis approach, Flavahan et al. [19] demonstrate that deficiency of CTCF binding at a particular domain boundary enables an aberrant enhancer promoter interaction that lead to oncogene activation, which promotes glioma formation.

In mammals such as humans and mice, female cells contain a pair of X chromosomes. However epigenetic silencing inactivates one copy of X through major reorganization of its structure. Interestingly, the mechanism of how certain genes can escape X inactivation was unknown until recently. Giorgetti et al. [23] studied X chromosome inactivation and how certain genes escape this process using gene expression integration with chromatin interactions (using Hi-C) and accessibility (using ATAC-seq). They also performed their integrative analysis in an allele-specific framework. They demonstrated that TAD formations are tightly associated with gene expression patterns only seen in certain active genes of the inactive X chromosome. Integration of RNA-seq, open chromatin regions and Hi-C data also highlighted clusters of genes that share patterns of accessibility, transcription and interaction that correlated with escape from X inactivation, as well as formation of TAD-like structures that encompass those regions.

The brief examples above demonstrate the power of integrative analysis in discovering new biology from complex datasets. In each of these situations, examining an individual data layer would not have provided the information needed to understand the complex system under study. All integrative methods (such as those described in combining Hi-C, ATAC-seq, ChIP-seq and RNA-seq data) have a number of limitations. Moreover, dimensionality issues arise from choosing a suitable measure of describing pairs of regions, i.e. use of two-dimensional data represented by Hi-C with combinations of one-dimensional data layers from ChIP-seq and RNA-seq. The most important limitation is the resolution of the data and sequence depth of each data type. Normalisation between each sample within the same data type is difficult especially when the data is obtained from multiple sources. Although RNA-seq is quite well studied in terms of normalisation between datasets, there is no established method for normalising ChIP-seq datasets. Hi-C data proves to be equally difficult due to the fledgling nature of the field.

5 Conclusions

Biomedical data integration is a complex and broad field and many different types of integrative approaches exist. Whilst an exhaustive comparison is not possible, we attempt to give an overview of integrative activities in this chapter at different technological and biological scales, from large and specialised data resources to statistical and computational integrative methods. We also provide examples of how combining two different biological layers can give insight into their joint influence and shed light on complex phenotypes in both normal and pathological situations.

References

1. Bader GD, Cary MP, Sander C (2006) Pathguide: a pathway resource list. Nucleic Acids Res 34:D504–D506. https://doi.org/10.1093/nar/gkj126
2. Bednar J, Horowitz RA, Grigoryev SA et al (1998) Nucleosomes, linker DNA, and linker histone form a unique structural motif that directs the higher-order folding and compaction of chromatin. Proc Natl Acad Sci U S A 95:14173–14178. https://doi.org/10.1073/pnas.95.24.14173
3. Berners-Lee T. (2006) Linked Data Design Issues. http://www.w3.org/DesignIssues/LinkedData.html. Accessed 30 June 2017
4. Benson DA, Cavanaugh M, Clark K et al (2017) GenBank. Nucleic Acids Res 45:D37–D42. https://doi.org/10.1093/nar/gkw1070
5. BioMart (2009) https://www.biomart.org. Accessed 30 June 2017
6. Biosharing (2016) https://biosharing.org. Accessed 30 June 2017
7. Brazma A (2009) Minimum information about a microarray experiment (MIAME)–successes, failures, challenges. SciWorld J 9:420–423. https://doi.org/10.1100/tsw.2009.57
8. Brown PO, Botstein D (1999) Exploring the new world of the genome with DNA microarrays. Nat Genet 21:33–37. https://doi.org/10.1038/4462
9. Cairns J (2012) Rcade: a tool for integrating a count-based ChIP-seq analysis with differential expression summary data. R package version 1.16.0
10. Casper J, Zweig AS, Villarreal C et al (2017) The UCSC Genome browser database: 2018 update. Nucleic Acids Res. https://doi.org/10.1093/nar/gkx1020
11. Chen H, Yu T, Chen JY (2013) Semantic web meets integrative biology: a survey. Brief Bioinform 14:109–125. https://doi.org/10.1093/bib/bbs014
12. Ching T, Huang S, Garmire LX (2014) Power analysis and sample size estimation for RNA-Seq differential expression. RNA 20:1684–1696. https://doi.org/10.1261/rna.046011.114
13. Cremer T, Cremer C (2001) Chromosome territories, nuclear architecture and gene regulation in mammalian cells. Nat Rev Genet 2:292–301. https://doi.org/10.1038/35066075
14. Crowdflower (2016) Crowdflower Data Science Report 2016. http://visit.crowdflower.com/rs/416-ZBE-142/images/CrowdFlower_DataScienceReport_2016.pdf. Accessed 30 June 2017
15. Dekker J, Mirny L (2016) The 3D genome as moderator of chromosomal communication. Cell 164:1110–1121. https://doi.org/10.1016/j.cell.2016.02.007
16. Durinck S, Spellman PT, Birney E, Huber W (2009) Mapping identifiers for the integration of genomic datasets with the R/Bioconductor package biomaRt. Nat Protoc 4:1184–1191. https://doi.org/10.1038/nprot.2009.97
17. Ernst J, Kellis M (2012) ChromHMM: automating chromatin-state discovery and characterization. Nat Methods 9:215–216. https://doi.org/10.1038/nmeth.1906
18. Fillbrunn A, Dietz C, Pfeuffer J et al (2017) KNIME for reproducible cross-domain analysis of life science data. J Biotechnol 261:149–156. https://doi.org/10.1016/j.jbiotec.2017.07.028
19. Flavahan WA, Drier Y, Liau BB et al (2016) Insulator dysfunction and oncogene activation in IDH mutant gliomas. Nature 529:110–114. https://doi.org/10.1038/nature16490
20. Functional Genomics Data Society (2010) http://fged.org. Accessed 30 June 2017

21. Galperin MY, Fernández-Suárez XM, Rigden DJ (2017) The 24th annual nucleic acids research database issue: a look back and upcoming changes. Nucleic Acids Res 45:5627. https://doi.org/10.1093/nar/gkx021

22. Giardine B, Riemer C, Hardison RC et al (2005) Galaxy: a platform for interactive large-scale genome analysis. Genome Res 15:1451–1455. https://doi.org/10.1101/gr.4086505

23. Giorgetti L, Lajoie BR, Carter AC et al (2016) Structural organization of the inactive X chromosome in the mouse. Nature 535:575–579. https://doi.org/10.1038/nature18589

24. Gligorijević V, Malod-Dognin N, Pržulj N (2016) Integrative methods for analyzing big data in precision medicine. Proteomics 16:741–758. https://doi.org/10.1002/pmic.201500396

25. Goble C, Stevens R (2008) State of the nation in data integration for bioinformatics. J Biomed Inform 41:687–693. https://doi.org/10.1016/j.jbi.2008.01.008

26. Henry VJ, Bandrowski AE, Pepin A-S et al (2014) OMICtools: an informative directory for multi-omic data analysis. Database (Oxford). https://doi.org/10.1093/database/bau069

27. Hoffman MM, Buske OJ, Wang J et al (2012) Unsupervised pattern discovery in human chromatin structure through genomic segmentation. Nat Methods 9:473–476. https://doi.org/10.1038/nmeth.1937

28. Hood L, Rowen L (2013) The Human Genome Project: big science transforms biology and medicine. Genome Med 5:79. https://doi.org/10.1186/gm483

29. Horbach SPJM, Halffman W (2017) The ghosts of HeLa: how cell line misidentification contaminates the scientific literature. PLoS ONE 12:e0186281. https://doi.org/10.1371/journal.pone.0186281

30. Hull D, Wolstencroft K, Stevens R et al (2006) Taverna: a tool for building and running workflows of services. Nucleic Acids Res 34:W729–W732. https://doi.org/10.1093/nar/gkl320

31. Illumina Press Release (2017) https://www.illumina.com/company/news-center/press-releases/press-release-details.html%3Fnewsid%3D2236383

32. Jenkinson AM, Albrecht M, Birney E et al (2008) Integrating biological data–the distributed annotation system. BMC Bioinform 9(Suppl 8):S3. https://doi.org/10.1186/1471-2105-9-S8-S3

33. Kalderimis A, Lyne R, Butano D et al (2014) InterMine: extensive web services for modern biology. Nucleic Acids Res 42:W468–W472. https://doi.org/10.1093/nar/gku301

34. Kirschner K, Samarajiwa SA, Cairns JM et al (2015) Phenotype specific analyses reveal distinct regulatory mechanism for chronically activated p53. PLoS Genet 11:e1005053. https://doi.org/10.1371/journal.pgen.1005053

35. Landfors M, Philip P, Rydén P, Stenberg P (2011) Normalization of high dimensional genomics data where the distribution of the altered variables is skewed. PLoS ONE 6:e27942. https://doi.org/10.1371/journal.pone.0027942

36. Leek JT (2014) svaseq: removing batch effects and other unwanted noise from sequencing data. Nucleic Acids Res. https://doi.org/10.1093/nar/gku864

37. Lieberman-Aiden E, van Berkum NL, Williams L et al (2009) Comprehensive mapping of long-range interactions reveals folding principles of the human genome. Science 326:289–293. https://doi.org/10.1126/science.1181369

38. Love MI, Huber W, Anders S (2014) Moderated estimation of fold change and dispersion for RNA-seq data with DESeq2. Genome Biol 15:550. https://doi.org/10.1186/s13059-014-0550-8

39. Luger K, Dechassa ML, Tremethick DJ (2012) New insights into nucleosome and chromatin structure: an ordered state or a disordered affair? Nat Rev Mol Cell Biol 13:436–447. https://doi.org/10.1038/nrm3382

40. Mammana A, Chung H-R (2015) Chromatin segmentation based on a probabilistic model for read counts explains a large portion of the epigenome. Genome Biol 16:151. https://doi.org/10.1186/s13059-015-0708-z

41. Martínez-Bartolomé S, Binz P-A, Albar JP (2014) The minimal information about a proteomics experiment (MIAPE) from the proteomics standards initiative. Methods Mol Biol 1072:765–780. https://doi.org/10.1007/978-1-62703-631-3_53

42. McQuilton P, Gonzalez-Beltran A, Rocca-Serra P et al (2016) BioSharing: curated and crowd-sourced metadata standards, databases and data policies in the life sciences. Database (Oxford). https://doi.org/10.1093/database/baw075
43. Merali Z, Giles J (2005) Databases in peril. Nature 435:1010–1011. https://doi.org/10.1038/4351010a
44. Morgan M, Carlson M, Tenenbaum D and Arora S (2017). AnnotationHub: Client to access AnnotationHub resources. R package version 2.6.5
45. National Centre for Biotechnology Information (1988) Bethesda (MD): National Library of Medicine (US), https://www.ncbi.nlm.nih.gov/NLM. Accessed 30 June 2017 (NCBI)
46. OmicTools (2014), https://omictools.com/. Accessed 30 June 2017
47. Pasquier C (2008) Biological data integration using semantic web technologies. Biochimie 90:584–594. https://doi.org/10.1016/j.biochi.2008.02.007
48. Pearson H (2001) Biology's name game. Nature 411:631–632. https://doi.org/10.1038/35079694
49. Pepke S, Wold B, Mortazavi A (2009) Computation for ChIP-seq and RNA-seq studies. Nat Methods 6:S22–S32. https://doi.org/10.1038/nmeth.1371
50. Pathguide: The pathway resource list (2006) TP53 knowledge based network models. http://www.pathguide.org. Accessed 30 June 2017
51. Robertson G, Hirst M, Bainbridge M et al (2007) Genome-wide profiles of STAT1 DNA association using chromatin immunoprecipitation and massively parallel sequencing. Nat Methods 4:651–657. https://doi.org/10.1038/nmeth1068
52. Robinson MD, McCarthy DJ, Smyth GK (2010) edgeR: a Bioconductor package for differential expression analysis of digital gene expression data. Bioinformatics 26:139–140. https://doi.org/10.1093/bioinformatics/btp616
53. Samarajiwa SA (2015) TP53 knowledge-based network models. http://australian-systemsbiology.org/tp53/. Accessed 30 June 2017
54. Samarajiwa SA, Forster S, Auchettl K, Hertzog PJ (2009) INTERFEROME: the database of interferon regulated genes. Nucleic Acids Res 37:D852–D857. https://doi.org/10.1093/nar/gkn732
55. Sawyer IA, Dundr M (2017) Chromatin loops and causality loops: the influence of RNA upon spatial nuclear architecture. Chromosoma 1–17. https://doi.org/10.1007/s00412-017-0632-y
56. Schadt EE, Linderman MD, Sorenson J et al (2010) Computational solutions to large-scale data management and analysis. Nat Rev Genet 11:647–657. https://doi.org/10.1038/nrg2857
57. Smedley D, Haider S, Durinck S et al (2015) The BioMart community portal: an innovative alternative to large, centralized data repositories. Nucleic Acids Res 43:W589–W598. https://doi.org/10.1093/nar/gkv350
58. Stein L (2002) Creating a bioinformatics nation. Nature 417:119–120. https://doi.org/10.1038/417119a
59. Stephens ZD, Lee SY, Faghri F et al (2015) Big data: astronomical or genomical? PLoS Biol 13:e1002195. https://doi.org/10.1371/journal.pbio.1002195
60. Taylor CF, Field D, Sansone S-A et al (2008) Promoting coherent minimum reporting guidelines for biological and biomedical investigations: the MIBBI project. Nat Biotechnol 26:889–896. https://doi.org/10.1038/nbt.1411
61. Wang S, Sun H, Ma J et al (2013) Target analysis by integration of transcriptome and ChIP-seq data with BETA. Nat Protoc 8:2502–2515. https://doi.org/10.1038/nprot.2013.150
62. Yates B, Braschi B, Gray KA et al (2017) Genenames.org: the HGNC and VGNC resources in 2017. Nucleic Acids Res 45:D619–D625. https://doi.org/10.1093/nar/gkw1033
63. Yu L, Fernandez S, Brock G (2017) Power analysis for RNA-Seq differential expression studies. BMC Bioinformatics 18:234. https://doi.org/10.1186/s12859-017-1648-2